Hematology and Immunology

Quality in Laboratory Diagnosis

Diagnostic Standards of Care

MICHAEL LAPOSATA, MD, PHD
Series Editor

Coagulation Disorders
Quality in Laboratory Diagnosis
Michael Laposata, MD, PhD

Clinical Microbiology
Quality in Laboratory Diagnosis
Charles W. Stratton, MD

Laboratory Management
Quality in Laboratory Diagnosis
Candis A. Kinkus

Transfusion Medicine
Quality in Laboratory Diagnosis
Quentin G. Eichbaum, MD, PhD, MPH, MFA, FCAP
Garrett S. Booth, MD, MS
Pampee P. Young, MD, PhD

Clinical Chemistry
Quality in Laboratory Diagnosis
James H. Nichols, PhD, DABCC, FACB
Carol A. Rauch, MD, PhD, FCAP

Hematology and Immunology
Quality in Laboratory Diagnosis
Adam C. Seegmiller, MD, PhD
Mary Ann Thompson, MD, PhD

Diagnostic Standards of Care Series

Hematology and Immunology
Quality in Laboratory Diagnosis

Adam C. Seegmiller, MD, PhD
Assistant Professor of Pathology, Microbiology, and Immunology
Director of Hematopathology
Vanderbilt University School of Medicine
Medical Director of Hematopathology and Immunopathology
Vanderbilt University Hospital
Nashville, Tennessee

Mary Ann Thompson, MD, PhD
Associate Professor of Pathology, Microbiology, and Immunology
Vanderbilt University School of Medicine
Medical Director of Hematology
Vanderbilt University Hospital
Nashville, Tennessee

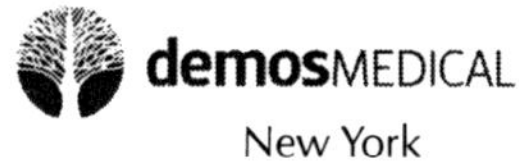

New York

Visit our website at www.demosmedical.com

ISBN: 978-1-62070-033-4
e-book ISBN: 978-1-61705-192-0

Acquisitions Editor: Richard Winters
Compositor: S4Carlisle Publishing Services

Medicine is an ever-changing science. Research and clinical experience are continually expanding our knowledge, in particular our understanding of proper treatment and drug therapy. The authors, editors, and publisher have made every effort to ensure that all information in this book is in accordance with the state of knowledge at the time of production of the book. Nevertheless, the authors, editors, and publisher are not responsible for errors or omissions or for any consequences from application of the information in this book and make no warranty, expressed or implied, with respect to the contents of the publication. Every reader should examine carefully the package inserts accompanying each drug and should carefully check whether the dosage schedules mentioned therein or the contraindications stated by the manufacturer differ from the statements made in this book. Such examination is particularly important with drugs that are either rarely used or have been newly released on the market.

Library of Congress Cataloging-in-Publication Data

Seegmiller, Adam C., author.
Hematology and immunology : quality in laboratory diagnosis / Adam C. Seegmiller, Mary Ann Thompson.
    p. ; cm. — (Diagnostic standards of care series)
  Includes bibliographical references and index.
  ISBN-13: 978-1-62070-033-4
  ISBN-10: 1-62070-033-6
  ISBN-13: 978-1-61705-192-0 (e-book)
  I. Thompson, Mary Ann (Professor of pathology, microbiology and immunology), author.
II. Title.   III. Series: Diagnostic standards of care.
  [DNLM: 1. Hematologic Tests—Case Reports.   2. Immunologic Tests—Case Reports.   3. Diagnostic Errors—Case Reports.   4. Medical Errors—Case Reports. QY 400]
  RB46.5
  616.07'56—dc23

2013048120

Printed in the United States of America by Gasch Printing.
14 15 16 17 / 5 4 3 2 1

*To Paula, Ethan, Hannah, Levi, and
Benjamin, with love—A.C.S.*

*To my husband, Ron, and my son, Mark, for their
love and encouragement—M.A.T.*

Contents

Series Foreword

"Above all, do no harm." This frequently quoted admonition to health care providers is highly regarded, but despite that, there are few books, if any, that focus primarily on how to avoid harming patients by learning from the mistakes of others.

Would it not be of great benefit to patients if all health care providers were aware of the thrombotic consequences from heparin-induced thrombocytopenia before a patient's leg is amputated? The clinically significant, often lethal, thrombotic events that occur in patients who develop heparin-induced thrombocytopenia would be greatly diminished if all health care providers appropriately monitored platelet counts in patients being treated with intravenous unfractionated heparin.

It was a desire to learn from the mistakes of others that led to the concept for this series of books on diagnostic standards of care. As the test menu in the clinical laboratory has enlarged in size and complexity, errors in selection of tests and errors in the interpretation of test results have become commonplace, and these mistakes can result in poor patient outcomes. This series of books on diagnostic standards of care in coagulation, microbiology, transfusion medicine, hematology, clinical chemistry, immunology, and laboratory management are all organized in a similar fashion. Clinical errors, and accompanying cases to illustrate each error, are presented within all of the chapters in several discrete categories: errors in test selection, errors in result interpretation, other errors, and diagnostic controversies. Each chapter concludes with a summary list of the standards of care. The most common errors made by thousands of health care providers daily are the ones that have been selected for presentation in this series of books.

Practicing physicians ordering tests with which they are less familiar would benefit significantly by learning of the potential errors associated with ordering such tests and errors associated with interpreting an infrequently encountered test result. Medical trainees who are gaining clinical experience would benefit significantly by first understanding what not to do when it comes to ordering laboratory tests and interpreting test results from the clinical laboratory. Individuals working in the clinical laboratory would also benefit by learning of the common mistakes made by health care providers so that they are better able to provide helpful advice that would avert the damaging consequences of an error. Finally, laboratory managers and hospital administrators would benefit by having knowledge of test ordering mistakes to improve the efficiency of the clinical laboratory and avoid the cost of performing unnecessary tests.

If the errors described in this series of books could be greatly reduced, the savings to the health care system and the improvement in patient outcomes would be dramatic.

Michael Laposata, MD, PhD
Series Editor

Preface

Medical decisions that impact patient care rely on the results of laboratory tests to a greater extent than ever before. At the same time, there has been a marked expansion in the number and complexity of tests offered. Both of these developments are driven, in part, by a desire to personalize medicine, thereby tailoring diagnosis, prognosis, and therapy to each patient individually. If applied properly, these developments promise to improve the care of patients. However, they also bring with them more opportunities to misapply and misinterpret laboratory tests, the risk and consequences of which increase with test number and complexity.

These challenges are particularly acute in the areas of hematology and immunology. Hematology tests are among the most common tests ordered by physicians. The routine complete blood count (CBC) is ordered and interpreted daily by many physicians of every specialty. Consequently, many thousands of important decisions that impact patient care hinge on the proper interpretation and application of these and related tests every single day. Despite its routine use, the CBC, red blood cell (RBC) indices, and white cell differential counts can be complex to interpret. They are fraught with potential pitfalls, which, if not recognized and understood, can lead to both missed and inappropriate diagnoses and therapies.

Immunology testing brings a related but distinct set of challenges. Serologic testing can be immensely helpful in diagnosing infectious and autoimmune diseases. However, these tests have limitations that must be recognized. If the tests are interpreted too broadly or out of context with patients' clinical findings, inappropriate diagnoses can be made, leading to unnecessary and potentially harmful treatment.

The case studies in this book are a reflection of our collective years of experience with these tests, involving implementation, quality control, and result interpretation. We have personally witnessed many of the errors described and their consequences, and we are eager to help others learn the important lessons taught by the errors.

It is our hope that this book, along with its companion volumes, will serve as an essential resource to pathologists, laboratorians, and clinicians, in the proper application and interpretation of laboratory tests, preventing errors, and improving the care of the patients to whom we devote our daily efforts.

Adam C. Seegmiller, MD, PhD
Mary Ann Thompson, MD, PhD

Acknowledgments

We are indebted to our teachers, mentors, and colleagues in pathology and laboratory medicine, who have broadened our experience through teaching and sharing. In particular, we thank Dr. Thomas McCurley, who graciously shared his decades of experience in hematopathology and immunology and suggested a number of the cases in this book. We also thank Dr. Michael Laposata, whose invitation, inspiration, and encouragement were essential to the conception and completion of this volume.

I
HEMATOLOGY

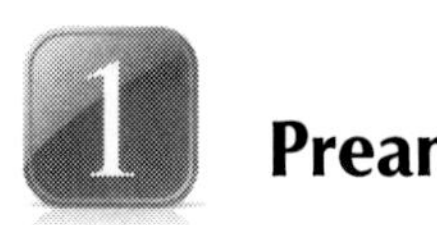 **Preanalytical Errors**

OVERVIEW

Hematology tests are sensitive to errors in specimen collection and handling. Samples collected for complete blood counts (CBCs) and peripheral blood smears should be collected from a peripheral vein, when possible, and transferred into an ethylenediaminetetraacetic acid (EDTA; lavender top) tube, following standard collection protocols, and processed in a timely fashion. Improper collection and/or handling can lead to significant errors in hematology results.

Case with Error

A 35-year-old woman presents to her primary care physician for an annual health examination. The physician orders routine laboratory studies, including a CBC. The nurse has difficulty collecting the sample and only fills the tube half-way. Results are as follows:

	Result	**Reference Range**
WBC	$7.1 \times 10^3/\mu L$	$3.9\text{--}10.7 \times 10^3/\mu L$
Hgb	13.5 g/dL	11.8–16.0 g/dL
Hematocrit	33.1%	36.1%–44.3%
Platelets	$302 \times 10^3/\mu L$	$135\text{--}371 \times 10^3/\mu L$
RBC	$4.6 \times 10^6/\mu L$	$4.0\text{--}5.5 \times 10^6/\mu L$
MCV	72 fL	81–98 fL
RDW	16.2%	11.1%–14.3%

Abbreviations: Hgb, hemoglobin; MCV, mean cell volume; RBC, red blood cells; RDW, red blood cell distribution width; WBC, white blood cell count.

The clinician interprets these results as indicating microcytic anemia. She calls the patient for a return appointment to collect iron studies. However, a repeat CBC is normal.

Explanation and Consequences

EDTA is the anticoagulant of choice for routine CBCs. However, the results of the tests are sensitive to EDTA concentrations. If the collection tube is not completely filled with blood, as in this case, the concentration of EDTA will be excessively high. Under these conditions, the red blood cells (RBCs) often shrink and may take on a crenated appearance on blood smear. As a result, the mean cell volume (MCV) measured by an automated analyzer will be falsely low. In addition, the hematocrit, which is calculated from the MCV and RBC count, will also be low.

One important clue for the interpreting physician is the correlation between the hemoglobin and hematocrit values. In general, the hematocrit/hemoglobin ratio is approximately 3:1. In this case, there is a discrepancy between a normal hemoglobin and abnormal hematocrit, with a ratio of 2.5:1. This should have suggested to the physician that the result may be spurious. Proper collection and interpretation could have prevented an extra office visit and additional unnecessary testing.

Case with Error

A 35-year-old man presents to his primary care physician for a routine physical examination. He reports being in good health and exercises regularly with no difficulty. The physician orders a CBC, the results of which are shown below:

	Result	**Reference Range**
WBC	$2.8 \times 10^3/\mu L$	$3.9–10.7 \times 10^3/\mu L$
Hgb	8.7 g/dL	14.0–18.1 g/dL
Platelets	$78 \times 10^3/\mu L$	$135–371 \times 10^3/\mu L$
RBC	$2.9 \times 10^6/\mu L$	$4.0–5.5 \times 10^6/\mu L$
MCV	88 fL	81–98 fL
RDW	12.9%	11.1%–14.3%

Upon seeing the results, the physician is concerned that there has been some mistake, as the patient was completely asymptomatic. He calls the laboratory and asks them to confirm the result. A technologist retrieves the sample and notices a large clot at the bottom of the tube that was not initially observed.

Explanation and Consequences

Clotted samples will give spurious results for CBC analysis. The peripheral blood cellular elements are sequestered in the clot, which significantly reduces their numbers in the liquid portion of the sample that is tested. Consequently, clotted samples can exhibit reduced blood counts in any or all lineages. In this case, the error resulted in a false report of pancytopenia that caused significant concern with the physician.

Case with Error

A 44-year-old man is hospitalized for pancreatitis. A CBC is drawn at the time of admission. The results are as follows:

	Result	**Reference Range**
WBC	$22.8 \times 10^3/\mu L$	3.9–$10.7 \times 10^3/\mu L$
Hgb	21.3 g/dL	14.0–18.1 g/dL
Platelets	$271 \times 10^3/\mu L$	135–$371 \times 10^3/\mu L$
RBC	$4.6 \times 10^6/\mu L$	4.0–$5.5 \times 10^6/\mu L$
MCV	85 fL	81–98 fL
MCHC	38 g/dL	31–35 g/dL
RDW	13.7%	11.1%–14.3%

The admitting physician notes the combination of high hemoglobin concentration and leukocytosis and consults the hematology service to evaluate the patient for a myeloproliferative disease. The next morning, other laboratory studies are ordered, including lipid studies that show a triglyceride level of 2,251 mg/dL (normal <150 mg/dL).

Explanation and Consequences

The measurement of hemoglobin involves a colorimetric assay. Lipemia can interfere with this measurement because it increases the turbidity of the sample. The result is an artificial increase in hemoglobin levels. The lipemia should have been visually noted in the laboratory, but it was missed. Many modern hematology analyzers note inconsistencies in blood counts and flag them for further analysis. In those cases, the hemoglobin measurement can be manually corrected for the lipemia.

In this case, the WBC count was also elevated, likely due to the underlying pancreatitis. However, combined with the falsely high hemoglobin level, this combination raised suspicion for a myeloproliferative process, and prompted an unnecessary consult. The physician could have suspected interference because the RBC count remained normal, despite the marked increase in hemoglobin value. In addition, the mean corpuscular hemoglobin concentration (MCHC) is spuriously elevated in samples that are turbid due to lipemia.

Case with Error

A 67-year-old woman was admitted to the hospital for an orthopedic procedure. Prior to surgery, the anesthesiologist ordered a CBC, the results of which are shown below:

	Result	**Reference Range**
WBC	$5.9 \times 10^3/\mu L$	$3.9–10.7 \times 10^3/\mu L$
Hgb	14.1 g/dL	11.8–16.0 g/dL
Platelets	$259 \times 10^3/\mu L$	$135–371 \times 10^3/\mu L$
MCV	83 fL	81–98 fL

The following morning, the patient's surgeon ordered a postoperative CBC, which showed:

	Result	**Reference Range**
WBC	$4.2 \times 10^3/\mu L$	$3.9\text{--}10.7 \times 10^3/\mu L$
Hgb	8.9 g/dL	11.8–16.0 g/dL
Platelets	$223 \times 10^3/\mu L$	$135\text{--}371 \times 10^3/\mu L$
MCV	102 fL	81–98 fL

With this apparent significant decrease in hemoglobin, the surgeon is very concerned that there might be postoperative bleeding. He orders several imaging studies and additional laboratory tests, including type and cross in preparation for transfusion. However, these tests did not identify a source of bleeding. A repeat CBC in the afternoon shows a normal hemoglobin of 13.5 g/dL.

Explanation and Consequences

This is a case of mistaken patient identification for the first postoperative CBC. The most likely explanation is that the patient's specimen was either mislabeled or in some other way switched with the specimen of another patient that had significant anemia. This had important consequences for this patient's care, in that it raised concern for clinical complications that were not actually present. This led to a series of unnecessary additional tests.

An important concept in the handling of test results is the so-called "delta check." This is a comparison between a patient's current result and his or her most recent prior result. There are a number of legitimate medical reasons why a number of the CBC parameters change over time. However, a patient's MCV does not usually undergo significant changes in a short period of time. In this case, the difference in MCV between the two specimens (83 fL vs. 102 fL) should have immediately raised questions about specimen identification.

This should have prompted a simple repeat of the CBC, which would have identified the error prior to any additional evaluation.

Case with Error

A 34-year-old woman with a history of lupus presents to her rheumatologist for her regular check-up. Her disease has been well controlled, and the rheumatologist reassures her that she appears to be doing well. As a matter of routine, he orders a CBC with leukocyte differential. The next day, he receives the results, which are normal, except for a comment that states "3+ echinocytes." He calls the lab for clarification. They confirm the results and tell him that echinocytes are a common finding in uremia. Given the patient's history, he is concerned that he may have missed a significant change in her renal status. He calls the patient back for additional laboratory studies to evaluate renal function. They are all normal, and a repeat peripheral smear examination does not identify significant echinocytes.

Explanation and Consequences

RBC morphology can be a very helpful diagnostic tool. However, it is extremely sensitive to artifacts when peripheral smears are not well made. Among the most common of these artifacts is echinocyte formation. Echinocytes are misshapen RBCs, characterized by cytoplasmic projections evenly distributed around the surface of the cell. They are distinguished from acanthocytes by preservation of central pallor. This can be a genuine pathologic finding in conditions such as renal disease with uremia, liver disease, vitamin E deficiency, and pyruvate kinase deficiency, among others. However, much more commonly, they are a laboratory artifact caused by slowly dried or overly thick blood smears, delays in blood processing, excessive exposure to EDTA (usually due to low sample volume), or altered pH.

Investigation revealed that on the date of the patient's first sample, the laboratory's automated slide maker and stainer was not operational, and all the slides were being made manually. The abnormal morphology in this case was due to a poorly made blood smear. The slide maker was operational for a later sample, and the artifact was no longer present on a well-made smear. This error, however, resulted in an additional office visit and unnecessary testing for the patient.

Case with Error

A 22-year-old man presents to the emergency department after 5 days of abdominal pain and diarrhea. He is diagnosed with viral gastroenteritis and severe dehydration. He is immediately given intravenous fluids, and then blood is drawn for laboratory studies. A CBC shows the following results:

	Result	**Reference Range**
WBC	$2.8 \times 10^3/\mu L$	$3.9–10.7 \times 10^3/\mu L$
Hgb	8.9 g/dL	14.0–18.1 g/dL
Platelets	$121 \times 10^3/\mu L$	$135–371 \times 10^3/\mu L$
RBC	$3.2 \times 10^6/\mu L$	$4.0–5.5 \times 10^6/\mu L$
MCV	87 fL	81–98 fL
RDW	12.9%	11.1%–14.3%

Seeing these results, the emergency department physician immediately admits the patient and consults hematology for evaluation of pancytopenia. The patient is scheduled for a bone marrow biopsy the following day. However, a repeat CBC the next morning is completely normal. The biopsy is canceled and the patient is discharged.

Explanation and Consequences

The site of phlebotomy is an important preanalytical consideration for hematology testing. In this case, the blood was drawn from the same arm where the intravenous line was inserted and proximal to the insertion site. Consequently, the drawn blood was diluted by the intravenous fluid, and the blood counts were all reduced. The blood should have been drawn from the opposite arm, or at least drawn from a site distal to the intravenous line insertion site. This would have prevented the initial interpretation of pancytopenia, and the patient would not have been admitted. Fortunately, the error was identified on the results of a second CBC, and the bone marrow biopsy was averted.

STANDARDS OF CARE

- Two patient identifiers should be confirmed before phlebotomy to ensure that the blood is being drawn from the correct patient. Tubes should be promptly labeled before drawing blood from a subsequent patient. Delta checks should be used in the laboratory to identify potential patient identification errors.
- For CBC testing, blood should be drawn into an EDTA (lavender top) tube. The tube must be completely filled to ensure that the EDTA concentration is within normal limits. The blood should be well mixed after collection into the tube to prevent clot formation and transported to the laboratory in a timely fashion.
- If a patient is receiving intravenous fluids, blood samples should be drawn from the opposite arm and from a peripheral vein, whenever possible. If the same arm must be used, the blood should be drawn from a site distal to the intravenous line insertion site.
- Specimens sent for CBC measurements should be carefully scrutinized in the laboratory for visual changes. They should be rejected if there are visible clots or if there is discernible hemolysis or lipemia.
- The quality of a peripheral blood smear should be taken into consideration when evaluating blood cell morphology. Smears that are too thick, poorly smeared, or air dried can have red cell artifacts. These possibilities should be considered before reporting significant abnormalities in RBC morphology.

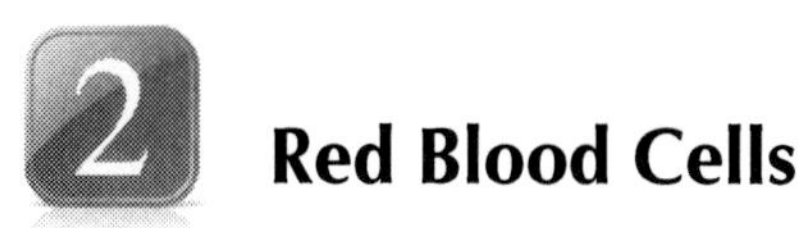

Red Blood Cells

ERRORS IN THE EVALUATION OF RED BLOOD CELL MORPHOLOGY

OVERVIEW

Red blood cells (RBCs) have a bi-concave shape that leads to a typical appearance on peripheral blood smear examination—round cells with central clearing or pallor that occupies approximately one third of the cell diameter. Variations in the shape of RBCs, so-called poikilocytosis, can occur in a number of clinical conditions, and, therefore, review of RBC morphology is an important diagnostic procedure. Many RBC morphology changes can be nonspecific, and their diagnostic value is dependent on the quality of the peripheral smear. Thus, RBC morphology, although very useful diagnostically, should not be relied upon as a sole diagnostic indicator for any condition.

Case with Error

A 27-year-old woman presents to the emergency department with fever and altered mental status. Complete blood count (CBC) results at the time of presentation are as follows:

	Result	**Reference Range**
WBC	$19.7 \times 10^3/\mu L$	$3.9 - 10.7 \times 10^3/\mu L$
Hgb	12.9 g/dL	11.8 − 16.0 g/dL
Platelets	$81 \times 10^3/\mu L$	$135 - 371 \times 10^3/\mu L$
RBC	$4.6 \times 10^6/\mu L$	$4.0 - 5.5 \times 10^6/\mu L$
MCV	82 fL	81 − 98 fL
RDW	15.2%	11.1% − 14.3%

The peripheral blood smear is reviewed by a technologist, who notes a number of what appear to be RBC fragments, small misshapen cells with residual central pallor. He reports "2+ schistocytes." The accompanying d-dimer and prothrombin time tests are in the normal range. Seeing these results, the physician is concerned about thrombotic thrombocytopenic purpura (TTP). He consults hematology and a plasma exchange procedure is begun as soon as possible.

Explanation and Consequences

Schistocyte is the term used to describe RBC fragments that appear as a consequence of microangiopathic hemolytic anemia, most commonly seen in TTP, disseminated intravascular coagulation, and hemolytic uremic syndrome. Schistocytes are generally small and misshapen with sharp angles or borders. They may be sickle-shaped, triangular, or "helmet"-shaped. The most definitive feature, however, is the absence of central pallor.

The poikilocytes in this case still had central pallor and, thus, should not have been categorized as schistocytes. Rather, they would best be described as "nonspecific poikilocytes." These cells can be seen in a number of conditions and are not specific for microangiopathic hemolytic anemias. In this case, the ADAMTS13 test, the definitive test for the diagnosis of TTP, was performed and found to be normal. Results from a lumbar puncture were consistent with viral meningitis.

In the absence of genuine schistocytes and with only moderate thrombocytopenia, a presumptive diagnosis of TTP should not have been rendered. The invasive and expensive plasma exchange procedure could have been avoided if the peripheral smear had been correctly interpreted.

Case with Error

A 7-year-old boy, an immigrant from Thailand, is admitted to the hospital for treatment of severe asthma. CBC results from the time of admission are as follows:

	Result	**Reference Range**
WBC	$6.3 \times 10^3/\mu L$	$5.0-14.5 \times 10^3/\mu L$
Hgb	13.2 g/dL	11.5−15.5 g/dL
Platelets	$328 \times 10^3/\mu L$	$250-450 \times 10^3/\mu L$
RBC	$5.0 \times 10^6/\mu L$	$4.0-5.2 \times 10^6/\mu L$
MCV	80 fL	75−95 fL
RDW	13.5%	11.1%−15.0%

The peripheral blood smear was reviewed by a technologist, who noted a significant number of target cells on the upper half, but not the lower half of the slide. Accordingly, she reported "2+ target cells." The admitting pediatrician notes this result and orders a hemoglobin electrophoresis study to rule out hemoglobinopathy.

Explanation and Consequences

Target cells are common in hemoglobinopathies, especially thalassemia and hemoglobin C disorders. Thus, the presence of target cells could prompt evaluation for hemoglobinopathy. However, it is important to rule out the possibility of an artifact. When blood smears are air dried, they may dry too slowly or unevenly. Under these conditions, there may be central precipitation of hemoglobin, causing artifactual target cells. In this case, the fact that the target cells were only seen on one part of the slide is strongly suggestive of artifact. Target cells due to hemoglobinopathy would be evenly distributed throughout the slide. In addition, there is no anemia, and the patient's RBC indices are normal. Recognition of this artifact could have prevented an unnecessary evaluation for hemoglobinopathy.

Case with Error

A 59-year-old man presents to his hematologist for a routine follow-up evaluation. He has a history of plasma cell myeloma that was treated with chemotherapy followed by autologous stem cell transplant. He has been in clinical remission for 6 months. CBC results are as follows:

	Result	Reference Range
WBC	$5.1 \times 10^3/\mu L$	$3.9-10.7 \times 10^3/\mu L$
Hgb	10.2 g/dL	11.8−16.0 g/dL
Platelets	$159 \times 10^3/\mu L$	$135-371 \times 10^3/\mu L$
RBC	$3.9 \times 10^6/\mu L$	$4.0-6.0 \times 10^6/\mu L$
MCV	95 fL	81−98 fL
RDW	15.4%	11.1%−14.3%

The peripheral blood smear was prepared by a manual method in the clinic. The hematologist reviews the slide and sees significant rouleaux formation. Concerned that this may be indicative of myeloma relapse, he orders serum and urine protein electrophoresis and schedules a bone marrow biopsy. However, neither protein electrophoresis study shows a monoclonal protein, and the bone marrow biopsy is negative for abnormal plasma cells.

Explanation and Consequences

Rouleaux formation is distinctive RBC aggregation that occurs in the presence of high levels of serum paraprotein, particularly monoclonal immunoglobulins in association with plasma cell neoplasms. In this way, it can be a helpful indicator of disease status. However, development of rouleaux formation is susceptible to artifacts. It is always seen in the thick part of a peripheral blood smear where the RBC concentration is greater. Genuine rouleaux formation, on the other hand, is also seen near the thin "feather edge" of the smear. Also, in genuine rouleaux formation the stacks of RBCs are arrayed in different directions, whereas in artifactual rouleaux formation the stacks are usually all arrayed in the same direction. In this case, the smear was poorly made and the leading edge was too thick. Consequently, there was artifactual rouleaux formation that was mistaken for evidence of recurrent disease. This led to additional unnecessary laboratory studies and invasive procedures.

STANDARDS OF CARE

▨ Peripheral blood smears should be made by an automated slide maker stainer, if possible, to ensure that smears are consistently well made and stained.

▨ If smears must be prepared manually, the persons preparing the smears should be subjected to rigorous training and appropriate quality control should be performed, because the ability to interpret the smear depends on its quality.

▨ Specific red cell morphologies should be reported as present using strict and specific criteria. For example, schistocytes should have sharp edges and angles with no central pallor, and target cells and echinocytes should be widely distributed on the smears rather than concentrated on a single part of the smear.

RECOMMENDED READING

Glassy EF, ed. *Color Atlas of Hematology: An Illustrated Field Guide Based on Proficiency Testing.* Northfield, IL: CAP Press; 1998.
Gulati G. *Blood Cell Morphology Grading Guide.* Chicago, IL: ASCP Press; 2009.

ERRORS IN THE DIAGNOSIS OF ANEMIA

OVERVIEW

Anemia is indicated by low hemoglobin and/or hematocrit and is categorized by mean cell volume (MCV) as microcytic, normocytic, or macrocytic. Distinguishing among causes of microcytic anemia is a common clinical problem. The differential diagnosis of microcytic anemia includes iron deficiency, anemia of chronic disease, and selected hemoglobinopathies, including thalassemia. These diagnoses can often be distinguished by a careful examination of the peripheral blood smear and examination of other RBC indices, including the RBC count, red cell distribution width (RDW), and reticulocyte hemoglobin (RetHe), among others. Diagnosis of iron deficiency anemia requires iron studies, including serum iron, total iron-binding capacity (TIBC), transferrin saturation (TSAT), and ferritin, the last of which is the most sensitive indicator.

Distinguishing the causes of microcytic anemia can be complicated when there are two or more different disorders at the same time, often leading to incorrect diagnoses. Thus, it is critical to understand how one disorder may be masked by the presence of another and how laboratory values are interpreted in these situations.

Case with Error

A 30-year-old female with a long history of anorexia nervosa is noted to have severe anemia by her primary care doctor. CBC values are as follows:

	Result	Reference Range
WBC	4.0 × 10³/μL	3.9−10.7 × 10³/μL
Hgb	6.6 g/dL	11.8−16.0 g/dL
Platelets	386 × 10³/μL	135−371 × 10³/μL
MCV	88 fL	81−98 fL

The primary care doctor counsels her on managing her anorexia and improving her diet. However, he does not recommend specific nutritional supplementation because he feels that her normal MCV rules out iron deficiency and vitamin B_{12} and folate deficiency. However, the patient continues to experience fatigue and weakness.

Explanation and Consequences

In this case, the primary care physician did not recognize the possibility of combined nutritional deficiencies, especially in a patient with a condition like anorexia, which predisposes to multiple dietary deficits. The physician assumed that neither iron deficiency, which normally causes microcytosis, nor vitamin B_{12} or folate deficiency, which normally causes macrocytosis, could be present in a patient with a normal MCV. This resulted in the failure to treat the underlying cause of the patient's anemia.

The patient saw another physician for a second opinion, who performed additional laboratory studies that showed:

	Result	**Reference Range**
Iron	21 μg/dL	50–150 μg/dL
TIBC	295 μg/dL	250–450 μg/dL
TSAT	7%	
Ferritin	18 ng/mL	20–300 ng/mL
RBC folate	413 ng/mL	342–786 ng/mL
Vitamin B_{12}	130 pg/mL	179–1132 pg/mL

With these data, her doctor initiated vitamin B_{12} and oral iron therapy, which resulted in significant improvement in the patient's symptoms.

Patients with poor nutrition can have coexisting nutritional deficiencies. These results can be misleading and cause a delay in diagnosis and definitive therapy of these deficiencies. Early recognition of vitamin B_{12} deficiency is particularly important, as it can lead to the subacute combined degeneration of the spinal cord, which may be only partially reversible with therapy.

Case with Error

A 20-month-old male is brought to his pediatrician by his parents, who recently emigrated from Thailand. They are concerned because he is not as active as his sister had been at this age. On physical examination, the pediatrician notes pale conjunctiva and a faint heart murmur. CBC values are as follows:

	Result	Reference Range
WBC	$11.7 \times 10^3/\mu L$	$6.0-17.0 \times 10^3/\mu L$
Hgb	8.0 g/dL	10.5−13.5 g/dL
Platelets	$354 \times 10^3/\mu L$	$135-371 \times 10^3/\mu L$
RBC	$4.9 \times 10^6/\mu L$	$3.7-5.3 \times 10^6/\mu L$
MCV	49 fL	70−86 fL
RDW	30.3%	11.5%−15.0%
Reticulocytes	1.6%	0.5%−1.8%

The pediatrician diagnoses iron deficiency anemia and prescribes oral iron supplements. At a 3-month return visit, the parents report little change in symptoms and a finger-stick hemoglobin is still low at 9.0 g/dL.

Explanation and Consequences

In this case, the pediatrician failed to recognize laboratory values indicative of thalassemia. He noted the low MCV and high RDW and incorrectly diagnosed iron deficiency anemia. While it is true that microcytosis and anisocytosis are hallmarks of iron deficiency, in this case the very low MCV (49 fL) and extremely high RDW (30.3%) are more typical for thalassemia. It is also important to consider the RBC count in evaluation of microcytic anemia. In iron deficiency, the Mentzer index (MCV/RBC) is almost always greater than 13, while an index lower than 13 is more typical of thalassemia. The index in this case was 10.

The patient was referred to a pediatric hematologist, who looked at a peripheral blood smear, which showed marked anisopoikilocytosis, schistocytes, target cells, and basophilic stippling, changes much more severe than are normally seen in iron deficiency anemia. Iron studies, including serum iron and ferritin, were normal. This prompted hemoglobin analysis (high-performance liquid chromatography [HPLC] and isoelectric focusing gel electrophoresis), which was consistent with α-thalassemia. This disorder is common in Southeast Asia, from where the patient's parents emigrated. The failure to recognize RBC indices characteristic of thalassemia, in favor of the more common diagnosis of iron deficiency, resulted in a delay in appropriate therapy for this patient.

Case with Error

A 2-year-old male, born of Laotian parents, presents with listlessness and pallor. Nutritional history reveals that the boy consumes four 8 oz. glasses of milk per day and eats little, if any, vegetables or fruit. The pediatrician suspects anemia and orders a CBC, the results of which are shown below:

	Result	**Reference Range**
WBC	$9.1 \times 10^3/\mu L$	$5.5 - 15.5 \times 10^3/\mu L$
Hgb	8.2 g/dL	11.5 − 15.5 g/dL
Platelets	$481 \times 10^3/\mu L$	$135 - 371 \times 10^3/\mu L$
RBC	$6.7 \times 10^6/\mu L$	$3.9 - 5.3 \times 10^6/\mu L$
MCV	45 fL	75 − 87 fL
RDW	27.3%	11.5% − 15.0%

As these values demonstrate a severe microcytic anemia, the primary care doctor appropriately follows up with iron studies, which show low serum iron, TSAT, and ferritin, consistent with iron deficiency. The patient is started on iron supplementation and the parents are told to limit his milk intake and introduce more fruits and vegetables. CBC at a follow-up visit shows:

	Results	**Reference Range**
WBC	$7.8 \times 10^3/\mu L$	$5.5 - 15.5 \times 10^3/\mu L$
Hgb	10.8 g/dL	11.5 - 15.5 g/dL
Platelets	$350 \times 10^3/\mu L$	$135 - 371 \times 10^3/\mu L$
RBC	$6.1 \times 10^6/\mu L$	$3.9 - 5.3 \times 10^6/\mu L$
MCV	65 fL	75 - 87 fL

The parents assure the physician that the iron supplements were taken as directed, despite the persistently abnormal hemoglobin and MCV. The physician thinks the patient may be resistant to oral iron therapy and recommends parenteral iron.

Explanation and Consequences

The primary care doctor noted microcytic anemia with a dietary history consistent with iron deficiency and appropriately ordered iron studies, which confirmed the diagnosis. However, an additional abnormality in the RBC indices was not appreciated, which explains the persistence of microcytosis, despite adequate iron therapy. In addition to low MCV, there was an elevated RBC count. The Mentzer index (MCV/RBC; described above) was 6.7, well below the cutoff value of 13 (values greater than 13 suggest iron deficiency anemia). This low index is more suggestive of hemoglobinopathy or thalassemia. In fact, subsequent hemoglobin analysis revealed 75% hemoglobin A (HbA), 23% hemoglobin E (HbE), and 2% hemoglobin F (HbF). Thus, in this case, iron deficiency was exacerbating an underlying HbE trait.

HbE is very common in Southeast Asia, particularly Cambodia, Laos, and Thailand. Individuals heterozygous for HbE (HbE trait) are asymptomatic, with mild microcytosis only. However, its presence can exacerbate the severity of iron deficiency anemia, as in this case. Proper interpretation of RBC indices would have led to recognition of this underlying disorder and would have prevented excessive iron therapy.

Case with Error

A 22-year-old African American female presents to the emergency department complaining of severe fatigue, bilateral hip pain, and a facial rash. She was told when she was a child that she had sickle cell trait and wonders if this pain could be related. The physician orders laboratory studies to determine whether she is anemic and also to rule out an infectious or rheumatologic explanation of her symptoms. CBC values are as follows:

	Results	**Reference Range**
WBC	$6.1 \times 10^3/\mu L$	$3.9-10.7 \times 10^3/\mu L$
Hgb	9.8 g/dL	11.8–16.0 g/dL
Platelets	$449 \times 10^3/\mu L$	$135-371 \times 10^3/\mu L$
RBC	$4.5 \times 10^6/\mu L$	$4.0-5.5 \times 10^6/\mu L$
MCV	72 fL	81–98 fL
Reticulocytes	1.0%	0.5%–1.8%
RetHe	28.8 pg	30.1–39.8 pg

Additional lab values indicate:

	Result	**Reference Range**
Ferritin	42 ng/mL	20–300 ng/mL
CRP	14.7 mg/L	<10 mg/L
ESR	30 mm/hr	0–10 mm/hr
ANA	Positive (1:160)	

The physician concludes that the patient has an autoimmune process, most likely lupus, as suggested by the symptoms and positive antinuclear antibody (ANA). He further concludes that the mild microcytic anemia is due to anemia of chronic disease associated with active inflammation, indicated by high C-reactive protein (CRP) and erythrocyte sedimentation rate (ESR). Iron deficiency is ruled out, the physician thinks, by the normal ferritin. Sickle cell trait is confirmed by HPLC, which shows HbA 57.9%, HbA2 3.8%, HbF <1%, and HbS 30.9%.

Immunosuppressive therapy for lupus is initiated. Over the next few months, the pain and rash improve, but the patient has persistent fatigue. Laboratory studies show no improvement in her microcytic anemia.

Explanation and Consequences

In this case, the physician inappropriately ruled out iron deficiency based upon a normal serum ferritin. Since the patient presented with active inflammation associated with lupus, it was concluded that the accompanying microcytic anemia was a result of anemia of chronic disease. However, there were three clues that suggested that the anemia was complicated by a component of iron deficiency. First, the RetHe was mildly reduced at 28.8 pg. This value, when low, is thought to be a marker for early iron deficiency. Second, the ferritin level was within the normal range, but the CRP and ESR were both elevated. Ferritin is an acute-phase reactant and is often elevated in patients with inflammatory disorders. Thus, in patients with inflammation, the ferritin alone is not an accurate measurement of iron load. Third, HPLC showed an HbS level of only 30.9%. In sickle cell trait, HbS generally makes up 35% to 40% of all hemoglobins. HbS of <33% is indicative of sickle cell trait with concomitant iron deficiency or α-thalassemia. If the correct diagnosis had been made initially, iron therapy could have been initiated to relieve the patient's symptoms related to anemia.

STANDARDS OF CARE

▧ The diagnosis of microcytic anemia should always include careful inspection of the peripheral blood smear and RBC indices, particularly the Mentzer index (MCV/RBC) to determine if thalassemia or other hemoglobinopathy should be considered in the differential diagnosis.

- Complete iron studies, including serum iron, TIBC, TSAT, and ferritin, should always be performed to confirm a presumptive diagnosis of iron deficiency as well as to establish a baseline for determining the efficacy of oral iron therapy. Although ferritin is the most sensitive indicator of iron deficiency, one should not rely on ferritin alone, as it can be falsely elevated in inflammatory states. RetHe should be reviewed when it is difficult to distinguish between iron deficiency and anemia of chronic disease.
- If microcytic anemia persists after appropriate oral iron supplementation, the patient should be screened for a hemoglobinopathy. This is especially important in immigrants from areas with a high incidence of hemoglobin mutations who may not have received newborn screening for these disorders.
- If HbS is <33% in a patient with sickle cell trait, a search for an additional cause of anemia, such as iron deficiency or α-thalassemia, must be initiated.
- In a patient with anemia and high suspicion of nutritional deficiency, a normal MCV should prompt examination of iron, vitamin B_{12}, and folate studies to rule out combined deficiencies of these dietary components.

RECOMMENDED READING

Bain BJ. *Haemoglobinopathy Diagnosis*. 2nd ed. Oxford, UK: Blackwell Publishing; 2006.

Glassy EF, ed. *Color Atlas of Hematology: An Illustrated Field Guide Based on Proficiency Testing*. Northfield, IL: CAP Press; 1998.

Hoyer JD, Kroft SH, eds. *Color Atlas of Hemoglobin Disorders: A Compendium Based on Proficiency Testing*. Northfield, IL: CAP Press; 2003.

Schoorl M, Schoorl M, Linssen J, et al. Efficacy of advanced discriminating algorithms for screening on iron-deficiency anemia and β-thalassemia trait. *Am J Clin Pathol*. 2012;138:300–304.

ERRORS IN INTERPRETATION OF RETICULOCYTE COUNT

OVERVIEW

> Reticulocytes are immature anucleate RBCs that circulate in the peripheral blood. The number of circulating reticulocytes is indicative of underlying erythropoiesis; that is, when erythropoiesis is stimulated, the number of circulating reticulocytes increases. Thus, the reticulocyte count can be used to differentiate anemias that are a result of RBC loss or destruction from anemias that are due to failure of marrow erythropoiesis.

Case with Error

A 33-year-old woman presents with increasing fatigue and weakness. The examining physician notes pallor and tachycardia and orders a CBC, the results of which are:

	Result	**Reference Range**
WBC	$4.1 \times 10^3/\mu L$	$3.9 - 10.7 \times 10^3/\mu L$
Hgb	7.9 g/dL	11.8 − 16.0 g/dL
Hematocrit	24%	36% − 49%
Platelets	$141 \times 10^3/\mu L$	$135 - 371 \times 10^3/\mu L$
RBC	$3.1 \times 10^6/\mu L$	$4.0 - 6.0 \times 10^6/\mu L$
MCV	88 fL	81 − 98 fL
RDW	14.5%	11.1% − 14.3%
Reticulocytes	0.8%	0.5% − 1.5%

Based on the normal reticulocyte count, the physician concluded that the bone marrow is responding adequately and that the anemia must be due to occult bleeding or hemolysis. Accordingly, additional laboratory tests, including direct antiglobulin test (DAT), lactate dehydrogenase (LDH), haptoglobin, and iron studies, were ordered. When they were found to be normal, a tagged erythrocyte study was ordered, but no source of bleeding was discovered.

Explanation and Consequences

In this case, the reticulocyte count was not interpreted in the context of the patient's anemia. The reticulocyte percentage can be misleading in an anemic patient because the denominator, the total RBC count, can be reduced and allows the reticulocyte percentage to be normal, although the absolute reticulocyte count is low. This issue can be addressed in two ways. First, if available, clinicians can use the absolute reticulocyte count to determine bone marrow response. This count is not falsely elevated in anemia. Second, if an absolute count is not available, a corrected reticulocyte count can be calculated. This is done by multiplying the reticulocyte percentage by the ratio of the patient's hematocrit to a standard hematocrit (taken as 45%). In this case, the corrected reticulocyte count is 0.4% (0.8% × [24%/45%] = 0.4%), which is low. Therefore, the patient most likely has anemia due to ineffective erythropoiesis.

Correctly calculated, this reticulocyte count may have led the clinician to consider a bone marrow failure syndrome. In fact, after no other explanation could be found, a bone marrow biopsy was performed, which showed a hypocellular marrow, consistent with early aplastic anemia. However, the error delayed this diagnosis and resulted in unnecessary and expensive diagnostic procedures.

STANDARDS OF CARE

- Absolute reticulocyte counts are preferable to reticulocyte percentages, when they are available. If percentages are used, they should be corrected for the degree of anemia, using the equation for the corrected reticulocyte count.

3 White Blood Cells

ERRORS IN THE EVALUATION OF GRANULOCYTIC LEUKOCYTOSIS

OVERVIEW

Granulocytic leukocytosis is an abnormality characterized by an elevated white blood cell (WBC) count in which the increase is predominantly due to increased granulocytes. These are usually neutrophils and precursors, but increased eosinophils may also be present. These findings may be accompanied by a "left shift," an increase in circulating neutrophil precursors, such as bands and metamyelocytes. Marked granulocytic leukocytosis with a left shift is often called a leukemoid reaction. These findings are a common reactive response to bacterial infections and physiologic stress. Similarly, eosinophilia can be caused be parasitic infections or allergic reactions. Both may occur in response to certain medications. However, similar findings are seen in neoplastic disorders, such as chronic myelogenous leukemia (CML) or eosinophilic leukemia. When a "left shift" is accompanied by nucleated red blood cells (RBCs), the pattern is called a leukoerythroblastic reaction and may indicate a space-filling or myelophthisic lesion, such as fibrosis or metastatic carcinoma. Care must be taken to recognize the features of these conditions so that a correct diagnosis is made and appropriate therapy initiated.

Case with Error

A 63-year-old man presents to the emergency department with bilateral lower extremity swelling and pain. The skin of both legs is red, tender, and swollen, with a large open lesion over the left tibia.

A clinical diagnosis of cellulitis is made. Complete blood count (CBC) values are as follows:

	Result	**Reference Range**
WBC	88 × 10³/μL	3.9–10.7 × 10³/μL
WBC differential		
Neutrophils	55%	35%–75%
Bands	5%	0%–2%
Metamyelocytes	6%	0%
Myelocytes	18%	0%
Promyelocytes	3%	0%
Blasts	1%	0%
Basophils	4%	0%–2%
Lymphocytes	8%	15%–49%
Hgb	9.5 g/dL	11.8–16.0 g/dL
Platelets	134 × 10³/μL	135–371 × 10³/μL

These abnormal results are attributed to the patient's infection and intravenous antibiotics are initiated. The patient is treated with a course of intravenous and oral antibiotics, and the cellulitis resolves. However, a repeat CBC at a follow-up clinic visit shows persistent leukocytosis with a similar differential and thrombocytopenia at 85 × 10³/μL. Careful physical examination reveals moderate splenomegaly. Peripheral blood is sent for cytogenetic analysis, which revealed an abnormal karyotype: 46,XY,t(9;22)(q34;q11). A bone marrow biopsy is performed and a diagnosis of CML, chronic phase is made.

Explanation and Consequences

This marked leukocytosis with left shift was inappropriately categorized as a leukemoid reaction to a severe infection. However, there were several clues that these abnormalities were not simply reactive.

First, the WBC count was much higher than is typical for reactive leukocytosis, which, while elevated, is usually less than 50 $\times$ 10³/µL. Also, the neutrophils were not only left-shifted with increased immature forms, but the distribution was abnormal, with a predominance of myelocytes and even rare blasts. Reactive neutrophilia can include a left shift, but the distribution tends to favor bands and metamyelocytes, with fewer of the more immature cells. The absolute basophil count was markedly elevated, calculated at 3.52 $\times$ 10³/µL (normal range 0.01–0.08 $\times$ 10³/µL), and careful examination would have revealed abnormal basophil morphology with decreased cytoplasmic granules. There was significant anemia and thrombocytopenia. Inflammation typically causes thrombocytosis, rather than thrombocytopenia, and usually does not depress the hemoglobin under 10 g/dL. Finally, the patient had splenomegaly, which was not recognized initially. These are all characteristics of CML that distinguish it from a leukemoid reaction.

Peripheral blood smear characteristics of leukemoid reaction and CML are:

Parameter	Leukemoid Reaction	CML
WBC	Usually <50 $\times$ 10³/µL	Usually >50 $\times$ 10³/µL
Toxic neutrophils	Present	Usually absent
Left shift	Present; mostly bands and metamyelocytes	Present with increased myelocytes; may include blasts
Basophilia	Absent	Present with atypical morphology
Nucleated RBCs	Absent	Present
Hemoglobin	Variable, usually >10 g/dL	Variable, may be <10 g/dL
Platelets	Variable, often increased	Variable, may be increased or decreased

Definitive diagnosis of CML is made by detection of the typical translocation, t(9;22)(q34q11), associated with this disorder. It can be detected by a number of diagnostic modalities, including karyotype, fluorescence in situ hybridization (FISH), and quantitative reverse transcription polymerase chain reaction (RT-PCR). This rearrangement causes fusion of the *BCR* and *ABL1* genes, resulting in a hybrid BCR-ABL1 protein that acts as a constitutively active tyrosine kinase, which drives granulocytic proliferation.

CML can be treated with a small-molecule tyrosine kinase inhibitor, imatinib. Delayed diagnosis increases the risk of morbidity and mortality associated with CML because, eventually, untreated CML typically progresses to an accelerated phase and then a blast phase, the latter of which is morphologically and clinically indistinguishable from acute leukemia. Timely diagnosis is important, because imatinib therapy is much less effective after disease progression.

Case with Error

A 35-year-old male presents to his physician complaining of shortness of breath, cough, and generalized pruritis. CBC results are as follows:

	Result	Reference Range
WBC	$8.4 \times 10^3/\mu L$	3.9–$10.7 \times 10^3/\mu L$
WBC differential		
Neutrophils	43%	35%–75%
Monocytes	5%	3.5%–12%
Eosinophils	31%	0.4%–7.5%
Basophils	1%	0%–2%
Lymphocytes	20%	15%–49%
Hgb	10.7 g/dL	11.8%–16.0 g/dL
Platelets	$115 \times 10^3/\mu L$	135–$371 \times 10^3/\mu L$

He recently has obtained two new pet dogs, and the physician thinks that the findings, including eosinophilia, are consistent with an allergic reaction. He prescribes an antihistamine, but the patient returns in 2 weeks with increased shortness of breath, rash, and a new onset of paresthesias in his hands and feet.

Explanation and Consequences

In this case, the physician failed to recognize the possibility of a chronic myeloproliferative neoplasm, such as hypereosinophilic syndrome or chronic eosinophilic leukemia, as a cause for eosinophilia. The approach was likely influenced by the relative rarity of these disorders compared with the more common causes of eosinophilia, such as allergic reactions, drug effects, and parasitic infections. However, in this case, the additional presence of anemia and mild thrombocytopenia, which is unusual in these reactive conditions, should have prompted an evaluation for a myeloproliferative process.

The patient was referred to a hematologist who reviewed his peripheral blood smear. He noted increased eosinophils, some of which had incomplete granulation, leaving bare areas of pale blue cytoplasm. The hematologist immediately sent blood for cytogenetic analysis, including FISH, which was positive for a FIP1L1-PDGFRA translocation involving FIP1L1 and the gene encoding platelet derived growth factor receptor-alpha. Both of these findings are consistent with a myeloproliferative neoplasm. He then ordered an echocardiogram, which demonstrated changes consistent with mild endomyocardial fibrosis.

The delay in diagnosis is significant in this case. Eosinophilic myeloproliferative diseases can cause permanent cardiac and/or pulmonary damage. Importantly, myeloproliferative disorders associated with FIP1L1-PDGFRA translocation or translocations involving PDGFRB (the gene encodiing platelet-derived growth factor receptor-beta) are exquisitely sensitive to low doses of the tyrosine kinase inhibitor imatinib, which causes rapid reduction of eosinophil counts.

STANDARDS OF CARE

A peripheral blood smear review should be performed for CBCs with leukocyte counts $>50 \times 10^3/\mu L$ or with automated WBC differential results indicating the presence of $>2\%$ immature granulocytes. Particular attention should be paid to the distribution of immature cells and the presence of increased atypical basophils and blasts.

▨ When analyzing CBC results, care should be taken to look for characteristics that are unusual for reactive neutrophilic leukocytosis before establishing this diagnosis. These may include anemia, thrombocytopenia or marked thrombocytosis, and basophilia, which could point to neoplastic disorders.

▨ There should be a low threshold for ordering a karyotype or FISH for *BCR/ABL1* on peripheral blood in a patient with neutrophilic leukocytosis. The presence of t(9;22) by either of these techniques is diagnostic of CML.

▨ FISH testing for translocations involving PDGFRA and PDGFRB should be performed for any patient that meets the criteria of hypereosinophilic syndrome, such as unexplained eosinophilia >1,500/μL, especially if there is evidence of eosinophil-mediated organ damage.

RECOMMENDED READING

Simon HU, Klion A. Therapeutic approaches to patients with hypereosinophilic syndromes. *Semin Hematol.* 2012;49:160–170.

Swerdlow SH, Campo E, Harris NL, et al., eds. *WHO Classification of Tumours of Haematopoietic and Lymphoid Tissues.* Lyon, France: IARC; 2008.

Tefferi A, Gotlib J, Pardanani A. Hypereosinophilic syndrome and clonal eosinophilia: point of care diagnostic algorithm and treatment update. *Mayo Clin Proc.* 2010;85:158–164.

ERRORS IN THE EVALUATION OF LYMPHOCYTIC LEUKOCYTOSIS

OVERVIEW

Lymphocytic leukocytosis is a normal reaction to a host of infectious (particularly viral or mycobacterial) and inflammatory conditions. Reactive lymphocytosis is often accompanied by a variety of changes in lymphocyte morphology. In addition, the number and morphology of lymphocytes vary with the patient's age. It is sometimes a challenge to distinguish these physiologic changes from those associated with chronic or acute lymphocytic leukemias. Careful attention to clinical history and peripheral blood smear morphology, and selective use of ancillary tests, such as flow cytometry, are crucial to making this important distinction.

Case with Error

A 1-month-old male is brought to an acute care clinic with a 3-day history of cough, poor feeding, lethargy, and posttussive emesis. Complete blood count (CBC) and differential are as follows:

	Result	**Reference Range**
WBC	44.1 × 10³/μL	4.0–14.6 × 10³/μL
WBC differential		
Neutrophils	32%	13%−33%
Monocytes	3%	4%−7%
Lymphocytes	65%	41%−71%
Hgb	12.1 g/dL	10.8−18.1 g/dL
Platelets	534 × 10³/μL	150–400 × 10³/μL

On the peripheral blood smear there are numerous atypical small lymphocytes with cleaved and slightly irregular nuclei. Seeing this morphology, the physician is concerned that this might be acute leukemia. He tells the parents that they should take their infant to the local pediatric hospital as quickly as possible for evaluation and potential bone marrow biopsy.

Explanation and Consequences

Evaluation of lymphocytosis in neonates can be difficult, especially in the setting of infection. Many viral and some bacterial infections can cause significant morphologic changes in lymphocytes, sometimes raising concern for leukemia. In this case, the patient was later shown to have a *Bordetella pertussis* infection by molecular studies for this organism. Pertussis is well known for causing lymphocytosis, often to levels $>11 \times 10^3/\mu L$. In rare cases, lymphocyte counts can be higher than $100 \times 10^3/\mu L$. Also, the lymphocytes are often morphologically atypical, with lobulated or cleaved nuclei, as in this case. In addition, the hemoglobin and platelet counts were normal and increased, respectively, while they are nearly always decreased in acute leukemia. The diagnostic error was not recognizing these features and overinterpreting what were reactive morphologic changes. If these had been properly recognized, a costly referral and leukemia evaluation could have been avoided.

While morphologic examination and clinical history are often adequate to suggest this diagnosis and to rule out leukemia, for difficult cases flow cytometry of the peripheral blood can be used to rule out acute leukemia. In addition, T cells from patients with pertussis will exhibit down-regulation of CD62L, a helpful marker since otherwise the T cells in these patients are a mix of CD4 and CD8 subsets with normal expression of CD7 and CD5. In addition, culture and molecular testing for *B. pertussis* is advised in infants with a worsening paroxysmal cough with an inspiratory whoop and/or posttussive vomiting.

Case with Error

A 49-year-old male presents with a several-day history of high-grade fever, malaise, myalgias, and mental status changes after he returned from a 1-week camping trip. He was admitted to the hospital where a CBC showed the following abnormal results:

	Result	**Reference Range**
WBC	$12.4 \times 10^3/\mu L$	3.9–$10.7 \times 10^3/\mu L$
WBC differential		
Neutrophils	20%	35%–75%
Lymphocytes	70%	15%–49%
Monocytes	10%	3.5%–12%
Hgb	9.0 g/dL	11.8–16.0 g/dL
Platelets	$30 \times 10^3/\mu L$	135–$371 \times 10^3/\mu L$

Review of the peripheral smear reveals some atypical lymphocytes. Examination of cerebrospinal fluid (CSF) shows increased lymphocytes and the patient has mild hepatosplenomegaly on imaging. Flow cytometry performed on the peripheral blood and CSF reveals increased gamma/delta T cells (27% in the peripheral blood). The clinician requests a hematology consult and schedules a bone marrow biopsy based on a concern for lymphoma, specifically gamma/delta hepatosplenic T-cell lymphoma.

Explanation and Consequences

In this case, the clinician was appropriately concerned about the possibility of lymphoma due to atypical lymphocytosis, predominantly composed of T cells expressing the gamma/delta T-cell receptor (gamma/delta T cells) that are normally seen at low concentrations in the peripheral blood. This was especially concerning in a patient with hepatosplenomegaly and clinical features that could be interpreted as "B symptoms." However, she did not consider the possibility of reactive or infectious causes of these symptoms.

In particular, the clinical features described here are also suggestive of infection by *Ehrlichia* species, a group of tick-borne Rickettsia that infect human leukocytes. Importantly, among the signs and symptoms of *Ehrlichia* infection is atypical lymphocytosis, which is caused by an increase in the number of reactive gamma/delta T cells. In fact, subsequent serologic tests were positive for IgM anti-*Ehrlichia* antibodies, indicating acute infection.

This error is of concern for two reasons. First, it delayed definitive therapy for the *Ehrlichia* infection. In this infection, treatment is most effective when initiated in the first 24–48 hours after diagnosis, and patients who are not treated with antibiotics promptly have a greater likelihood of severe disease or even death. In fact, the mortality rate among patients with symptoms severe enough to seek medical treatment is 1%–3%. Second, it led to an inappropriate referral and an unnecessary diagnostic procedure.

Case with Error

A 5-year-old male is brought to his pediatrician by his mother because she is concerned about several small lumps in his neck. She says that he had a sore throat 2 weeks ago and also that he has had some abdominal discomfort. Examination reveals bilateral enlarged lymph nodes and splenomegaly. The pediatrician obtains a CBC that shows:

	Result	**Reference Range**
WBC	$14.1 \times 10^3/\mu L$	$5.0–14.5 \times 10^3/\mu L$
WBC differential		
Neutrophils	25%	32%–54%
Lymphocytes	34%	28%–48%
Atypical lymphs	27%	N/A
Monocytes	10%	3%–6%
Eosinophils	3%	0%–3%
Basophils	1%	0%–1%
Hgb	12.4 mg/dL	11.5–15.5 mg/dL
Platelets	$110 \times 10^3/\mu L$	$250–450 \times 10^3/\mu L$

The medical technologist reviewing the smear contacts the pediatrician with concern about the possibility of lymphoma. She states that the lymphocytes are variably sized, but many are large with prominent nucleoli and deep basophilic cytoplasm. The pediatrician immediately refers the patient to a local children's hospital to be evaluated for lymphoma.

Explanation and Consequences

Not all atypical lymphocytes are neoplastic. In fact, patients with infectious diseases, particularly viral illnesses such as infectious mononucleosis, can exhibit reactive lymphocytes in the peripheral blood with markedly atypical morphology. They can have large, irregular nuclei, immature chromatin, prominent nucleoli, and/or dark basophilic cytoplasm. They may be sufficiently atypical to prompt concern for lymphoma, such as Burkitt lymphoma, or even acute leukemia. Thus, it is important to consider the clinical context and rule out common infectious diseases before raising concern for a less common neoplastic process.

Examination of the peripheral smear can also assist in the diagnosis. Reactive lymphocytes that arise in viral illness will exhibit variability in size, shape, nuclear chromatin, and color of the cytoplasm, whereas the neoplastic lymphocytes of leukemia or lymphoma tend to have a more uniform appearance. Also, the abundant cytoplasm of reactive lymphocytes, particularly in infectious mononucleosis, is often indented by surrounding erythrocytes, and the edges of the cytoplasm are often more intensely basophilic.

In this case, the error led to an unnecessary and expensive referral. At the children's hospital, an on-call hematologist recognized the characteristic morphologic signs on the peripheral smear as well as the clinical context. The hematologist ordered a monospot test, which was negative. However, because some young children have false-negative monospot tests, she ordered serologic tests for IgM and IgG antiviral capsid antigen (anti-VCA) antibodies, which were positive, indicating acute infectious mononucleosis.

Case with Error

A 2-year-old male is brought to his pediatrician by his mother due to 1 week of nausea, diarrhea, poor feeding, and lethargy. The pediatrician makes a presumptive diagnosis of viral gastroenteritis. As part of her evaluation she orders a CBC, the results of which are as follows:

	Result	**Reference Range**
WBC	$12.7 \times 10^3/\mu L$	$6.0–17.5 \times 10^3/\mu L$
WBC differential		
Neutrophils	20%	35%–80%
Lymphocytes	62%	50%–70%
Monocytes	8%	0%–10%
Blasts	8%	0%
Hgb	12.7 g/dL	9.4–13.0 g/dL
Platelets	$250 \times 10^3/\mu L$	$150–440 \times 10^3/\mu L$

The physician is alarmed by the presence of blasts on the automated differential and advises the mother to immediately take her son to the emergency department of the local children's hospital to be evaluated for acute leukemia.

Explanation and Consequences

Physicians are always appropriately concerned by a report of blasts in the peripheral blood, especially in children. However, in this case, the physician should have evaluated this result in the context of the complete clinical picture. It is important to recognize that blasts can be confused with normal circulating B-cell precursors, termed hematogones, by both automated hematology analyzers and human reviewers. Circulating hematogones are more common in young children, especially in reactive conditions such as infection. They are often confused for lymphoblasts because their nuclei can be slightly convoluted and the chromatin slightly more immature than normal lymphocytes. In especially difficult cases, flow cytometry can definitively distinguish between normal and neoplastic immature lymphocytes.

Another important feature to consider is the usual clinical context of acute leukemia. It almost always presents with anemia and thrombocytopenia, and their accompanying clinical sequelae. However, both the hemoglobin and the platelet count were normal in this case.

Upon presentation to the children's hospital, a peripheral blood smear was reviewed by a hematopathologist, who determined that, in fact, the so-called "blasts" were normal immature lymphocytes. This was confirmed by flow cytometry. Recognition of the clinical context and the possibility of over-calling blasts in this situation should have prompted the physician to do a more thorough evaluation prior to issuing what was ultimately an incorrect diagnosis, making an unnecessary referral, and unduly alarming the parents.

STANDARDS OF CARE

- Absolute lymphocytosis should prompt manual review of the peripheral blood smear to help distinguish a reactive from a neoplastic process. Particular care should be taken in young children, in whom normal immature lymphocytes may circulate.
- The differential diagnosis of atypical lymphocytosis should always include reactive and infectious conditions, such as pertussis, ehrlichiosis, and infectious mononucleosis. These conditions should be ruled out by a careful clinical history, physical examination, and appropriate laboratory testing prior to a diagnosis of or referral for leukemia or lymphoma.
- In difficult cases, flow cytometry should be used to help distinguish reactive lymphocytosis from leukemia or lymphoma.

RECOMMENDED READING

Caldwell CW, Everett ED, McDonald G, Yesus YW, Roland WE. Lymphocytosis of gamma/delta T cells in human ehrlichiosis. *Am J Clin Pathol.* 1995;103:761–766.

Gattens M, Morilla R, Bain BJ. Teaching cases from the Royal Marsden and St. Mary's Hospitals. Case 24: Striking lymphocytosis in a 2-year old girl. *Leuk Lymphoma.* 2004;45:851–852.

Glassy EF, ed. *Color Atlas of Hematology: An Illustrated Field Guide Based on Proficiency Testing.* Northfield, IL: CAP Press; 1998.

Hamilton KS, Standaert SM, Kinney MC. Characteristic peripheral blood findings in human ehrlichiosis. *Mod Pathol.* 2004;17:512–517.

Hudnall SD, Molina CP. Marked increase in L-selectin-negative T cells in neonatal pertussis. *Am J Clin Pathol.* 2000;114:35–40.

ERRORS IN THE DIAGNOSIS OF MYELODYSPLASIA

OVERVIEW

Myelodysplastic syndrome (MDS) is a clonal neoplasm of myeloid precursors characterized by peripheral cytopenias of myeloid, erythroid, and/or platelet lineages due to ineffective hematopoiesis. This leads to cytopenia-associated complications, including susceptibility to infection, anemia, and bleeding diathesis. Additionally, there is increased risk for the development of acute myeloid leukemia. Because peripheral blood and/or bone marrow elements generally exhibit morphologic dysplasia, diagnosis of MDS relies heavily on morphologic examination of peripheral blood and bone marrow aspirate smears. However, dysplasia is not a specific finding. It can be seen in a number of other disorders that exhibit clinical and laboratory findings similar to those of MDS, but for which the treatment and prognosis are much less severe. Thus, it becomes critical to accurately distinguish true MDS from its morphologic mimics.

Case with Error

A 58-year-old female presents to her primary care physician with complaints of increasing fatigue over the past 6 months. On physical examination, he notes pallor and tachycardia. This prompts him to order a complete blood count (CBC), which shows pancytopenia with macrocytic anemia, as follows:

	Result	**Reference Range**
WBC	$2.0 \times 10^3/\mu L$	$3.9-10.7 \times 10^3/\mu L$
Hgb	7.7 g/dL	11.8−16.0 g/dL
Platelets	$99 \times 10^3/\mu L$	$135-371 \times 10^3/\mu L$
MCV	124 fL	81−98 fL
Reticulocytes	1.2%	0.5%−1.8%

The patient is transfused with 2 units of packed red blood cells (RBCs) and referred to a hematologist. The hematologist reviews a peripheral blood smear that shows macrocytic anemia with large ovalocytes, anisocytosis, and rare hypersegmented neutrophils. Additional studies reveal vitamin B_{12} and RBC folate levels within normal ranges. Bone marrow biopsy reveals a markedly hypercellular marrow with marked erythroid and myeloid dysplasia, nucleus/cytoplasm dyssynchrony, giant metamyelocytes and bands, and cytoplasmic vacuoles in pronormoblasts. A diagnosis of low-grade MDS is rendered. The patient is followed closely and receives two additional RBC transfusions over the ensuing months.

Explanation and Consequences

In this case, megaloblastic anemia was misdiagnosed as a low-grade MDS. Megaloblastic anemia describes the hematologic findings that are associated with nutritional deficiencies of vitamin B_{12} and of folate. These findings, which include pancytopenia, hypercellular bone marrow with ineffective hematopoiesis, and marked morphologic dysplasia, can be remarkably similar to those of low-grade MDS. Recognizing this, the hematologist appropriately ordered vitamin B_{12} and RBC folate levels, both of which were normal. However, these findings were misleading in the context of recent RBC transfusion. The hematologist ordered RBC folate, presumably because it is a better reflection of folate stores and less susceptible to recent dietary changes. While this is true, RBC folate levels can be falsely elevated for up to several weeks after RBC transfusion due to the presence of donor erythrocytes. Thus, the patient's recent transfusion masked an underlying folate deficiency.

Several months later, the hematologist repeated the nutritional studies, including serum folate. In the absence of transfusion, both serum and RBC folate levels were low, indicating folate deficiency. A trial of folate supplementation resulted in marked improvement in clinical signs and symptoms and normalized the patient's CBC results (Hgb 12.3 mg/dL; MCV 93 fL). Proper use of the serum folate test at initial presentation would have prevented a costly and invasive bone marrow biopsy and the subsequent blood transfusions that the patient received.

Case with Error

A 34-year-old female presents to her primary care physician with weight loss, fatigue, and dizziness. Laboratory studies reveal anemia and leukopenia. Her physician treats her with iron and vitamin B_{12} supplements, but her blood cell counts continue to decrease, prompting referral to a hematologist. At the time of referral, CBC values are as follows:

	Result	**Reference Range**
WBC	$2.4 \times 10^3/\mu L$	$3.9 - 10.7 \times 10^3/\mu L$
Hgb	6.5 g/dL	11.8 − 16.0 g/dL
Platelets	$216 \times 10^3/\mu L$	$135 - 371 \times 10^3/\mu L$
MCV	103 fL	81 − 98 fL
Vitamin B_{12}	2011 pg/mL	179 − 1132 pg/mL
RBC folate	351 ng/mL	342 − 786 pg/mL

The hematologist performs a bone marrow biopsy that shows left-shifted myeloid maturation with prominent cytoplasmic vacuoles in approximately 20% of erythroid and myeloid precursors. A Prussian blue-stained aspirate smear shows scattered ringed sideroblasts. Based on this morphology and clinical history, a diagnosis of MDS is rendered. The patient is transfused and treatment with erythropoietin and azacitidine is initiated.

The patient is followed for 1 year, without consistent improvement in blood cell counts or symptoms. She gradually develops numbness and tingling in her toes that progress to loss of sensation in her lower extremities, weakness in legs and hands, and bilateral foot and wrist drop. She is finally referred for a stem cell transplant evaluation.

Explanation and Consequences

The physicians in this case did not recognize an uncommon but important cause of cytopenias with dysplasia. The stem cell transplant referral physician repeated the laboratory studies described above, but also ordered a serum copper level, which was 2 µg/dL (normal 80–155 µg/dL). The patient was given copper gluconate, after which her counts and symptoms improved. However, even after complete recovery of blood counts, she had persistent neurologic deficits.

Copper deficiency is a rare cause of anemia. As a key co-factor in iron metabolism, its absence leads to defects in hematopoiesis. Deficiency is often due to zinc overload, as zinc and copper compete for absorption in the proximal small bowl. Zinc excess may be due to excessive use of zinc supplements or ointments used for a variety of purposes or to environmental exposure. Copper deficiency can also be seen in patients with total parenteral hyperalimentation, intestinal malabsorption after gastrectomy, enteropathies, starvation, and Menkes syndrome.

Bone marrow aspirate smears in patients with copper deficiency have a distinctive appearance, with multiple cytoplasmic vacuoles present in both the myeloid precursors and erythroid precursors. There are also occasional ringed sideroblasts on iron stains and left-shifted myeloid maturation. These features overlap with those that can be seen in MDS, resulting in occasional misdiagnosis, as was seen in this case. If recognized, however, they can prompt an evaluation for copper deficiency.

There are several important consequences for missing the signs of copper deficiency in this case. First, the patient received an invasive bone marrow biopsy that was unnecessary. Second, the patient carried a false diagnosis of MDS and received unnecessary treatments for MDS and preventable transfusions. Third, the long-term sequelae of copper deficiency include neurologic deficits that may not be completely reversible. Thus, a timely and accurate diagnosis is necessary.

Case with Error

A 9-year-old male is brought to his pediatrician, complaining of shortness of breath and a persistent cough for 2 weeks. The pediatrician is concerned for pneumonia and performs a complete evaluation, including a CBC, which shows:

	Result	**Reference Range**
WBC	$9.7 \times 10^3/\mu L$	$3.9-10.7 \times 10^3/\mu L$
Hgb	13.3 g/dL	11.8−16.0 g/dL
Platelets	$362 \times 10^3/\mu L$	$135-371 \times 10^3/\mu L$
MCV	83 fL	81−98 fL

The results are flagged due to increased immature granulocytes (5%). Review of a peripheral blood smear reveals many dysplastic neutrophils with uniformly bi-lobed nuclei seen in almost all of the neutrophils. Concerned for MDS, the pediatrician refers the patient to hematology and a bone marrow biopsy is performed. However, other than the abnormal peripheral blood neutrophils, there is no evidence for myelodysplasia. Cytogenetic studies on the bone marrow show a normal male karyotype.

Explanation and Consequences

In this case, the physician receiving the report and the pathologist reviewing the blood smear did not recognize Pelger-Huet anomaly, an inherited condition in which most or all of the neutrophils are hypolobated, with only one lobe (in the homozygous form) or two lobes (the heterozygous form), instead of the normal three to five. This is a benign condition that usually has no additional clinical consequences.

While similar cells can also be seen in MDS (termed "pseudo-Pelger-Huet cells"), they usually only represent a subset of all neutrophils and tend to exhibit more nuclear heterogeneity, as well as other dysplastic features, such as hypogranular cytoplasm. In addition, pseudo-Pelger-Huet cells can be seen in infections, such as HIV, tuberculosis, and *Mycoplasma* pneumonia. Another important consideration is that patients with MDS have ineffective hematopoiesis by definition. Thus, suspicion for MDS should not arise in a patient with normal blood counts, as in this case.

The consequence of this error is that the patient received an unnecessary bone marrow biopsy and was unnecessarily subjected to the associated cost, pain, and potential complications of this invasive procedure. If appropriately recognized, the patient and his family could have been reassured that the abnormal findings were benign and carried no negative prognosis.

STANDARDS OF CARE

- A complete nutritional study should be performed when investigating any new-onset macrocytic anemia. These studies should include tests for vitamin B_{12}, serum and RBC folate, copper, and zinc. RBC folate levels should be obtained before RBC transfusion.
- Bone marrow biopsy should be avoided if there is evidence of nutritional deficiency. If a bone marrow biopsy is performed, it is important to recognize that nutritional deficiencies can cause profound morphologic dysplasia. Thus, these findings should not be used as sole evidence of MDS. In fact, cytogenetic abnormalities may transiently be present due to B_{12} or folate deficiency as well.
- Morphologic dysplasia, such as Pelger-Huet cells, can be caused by a number of conditions other than MDS. Thus, one should rule out inherited, infectious, inflammatory, and nutritional causes before rendering a definitive diagnosis of MDS.
- MDS is almost always associated with one or more cytopenias. Caution should be exercised in the evaluation for MDS if the patient has a normal or near-normal CBC. In many cases, a repeat CBC after a period of time should be performed before proceeding with an invasive procedure such as a bone marrow biopsy.

RECOMMENDED READING

Kjeldsberg CR, ed. *Practical Diagnosis of Hematologic Disorders, Benign Disorders*. 4th ed. Chicago, IL: ASCP Press; 2006.
Willis MS, Monaghan SA, Miller ML, et al. Zinc-induced copper deficiency: a report of three cases initially recognized on bone marrow examination. *Am J Clin Pathol*. 2005;123:125–131.

4 **Platelets**

ERRORS IN THE EVALUATION OF THROMBOCYTOPENIA

OVERVIEW

The differential diagnosis of thrombocytopenia is broad and can involve defects in both bone marrow production of platelets and peripheral destruction or consumption of platelets. In either case, thrombocytopenia can indicate a significant bleeding risk and may be a marker of a serious underlying disorder. For these reasons, an accurate platelet count is crucial to clinical decision making. However, spuriously low platelet counts occur due to both technical and physiologic causes. It is important to recognize these causes and rule them out by careful evaluation of a peripheral blood smear to prevent unnecessary procedures and incorrect diagnoses.

Case with Error Averted

A 50-year-old female presents for a routine annual examination. She is in her usual state of health, except that she complains of being more fatigued than usual. The physician performs a thorough physical examination and finds no abnormalities. He orders a routine CBC and is surprised when the laboratory calls to report a critical platelet count of $20 \times 10^3/\mu L$. He does not remember seeing bruising, petechiae, or other indications of thrombocytopenia on physical examination, but he calls the patient and schedules her to see a hematologist for a bone marrow biopsy later in the week.

The hematologist reviews the patient's peripheral blood smear and notes many platelet clumps. Based on this examination, she orders a repeat CBC for the patient's visit, specifying that it be drawn into a citrate tube (yellow top) rather than an ethylenediaminetetraacetic acid (EDTA) tube (purple top). Comparison of the two CBCs are shown below:

CBC Parameter	Draw #1: EDTA	Draw #2: Citrate
WBC	$10.8 \times 10^3/\mu L$	$6.8 \times 10^3/\mu L$
Hematocrit	39%	39%
Platelets	$20 \times 10^3/\mu L$	$182 \times 10^3/\mu L$

Seeing these results, the hematologist cancels the bone marrow examination and reassures the patient that her platelet count is normal.

Explanation and Consequences

In this case, the primary care physician failed to recognize the possibility of a decreased platelet count due to artifact rather than true thrombocytopenia. This resulted in an inappropriate referral and may have led to an unnecessary invasive procedure. Fortunately, this outcome was averted by the hematologist, who appropriately reviewed the peripheral smear and discovered the artifact.

This was a case of EDTA-dependent pseudothrombocytopenia, one of the most common causes of spuriously low platelet counts obtained from hematology analyzers. It has an estimated prevalence of 0.07%–0.2% of samples, but represents a significant percentage of patients from the average outpatient clinic who are referred for evaluation of thrombocytopenia. In certain patients with no particular demographic or clinical profile, the EDTA anticoagulant in the vacuum tube used for a CBC causes platelets to aggregate. Aggregation occurs quickly after exposure of the blood to EDTA, and is more evident at room temperature. Most blood samples from these patients will not exhibit platelet clumping if the blood is drawn into a tube with sodium citrate as an anticoagulant.

In this case, the hematologist appropriately recognized the possibility of platelet clumping as a cause of apparent thrombocytopenia in an otherwise healthy, asymptomatic patient. She correctly reviewed a peripheral blood smear to look for artifacts, such as platelet clumping. This artifact will be evident as aggregated platelet clumps found at the feather edge or along the side edges of the slide. Careful examination of the results from the hematology analyzer may also suggest platelet clumping. For example, the platelet size histogram may have a shoulder of what appear to be large platelets, and the white blood cells (WBCs) may be falsely elevated due to medium-size clumps being mistakenly counted as leukocytes.

Case with Error Averted

A 39-year-old female from Lebanon who presents with new onset of neuro-Behcet's syndrome is undergoing an initial evaluation by her rheumatologist. This included a CBC that generated the following results:

	Result	Reference Range
WBC	$5.1 \times 10^3/\mu L$	$3.9-10.7 \times 10^3/\mu L$
Hgb	14.8 g/dL	$11.8-16.0$ g/dL
Platelets	$80 \times 10^3/\mu L$	$135-371 \times 10^3/\mu L$

The rheumatologist was surprised by the thrombocytopenia and referred the patient to a hematologist, concerned that the patient needed treatment for concomitant idiopathic thrombocytopenic purpura (ITP).

The hematologist noted an absence of physical signs or symptoms typically associated with thrombocytopenia, such as a petechial or purpuric rash. Upon review of the peripheral smear, the hematologist noted that many neutrophils were encircled by adherent platelets and correctly concluded that the platelet count was low due to platelet satellitism. Thus, he was able to reassure the patient that the abnormal result was artifactual and that no intervention was required.

Explanation and Consequences

Similar to the previous case, the initial physician evaluating the patient did not consider artifact as a possible cause for the low platelet count, leading to an erroneous initial diagnosis of ITP. Fortunately, the patient avoided therapy for an inappropriate diagnosis because the hematologist reviewed the peripheral smear and noted evidence of platelet satellitism, another artifact that causes spuriously low platelet counts.

Platelet satellitism is a phenomenon in which platelets adhere to leukocytes, usually neutrophils. On Wright-stained peripheral blood smears, these platelets can be seen to encircle neutrophils. As they are adhered to leukocytes, these platelets are not detected by automated hematology analyzers, and the reported platelet count is reduced. One clue to this artifact is that the hematology analyzer may indicate an abnormal leukocyte distribution on the scattergram, as the neutrophils will appear too large with abnormal light scatter properties.

Usually, platelet satellitism is EDTA-related, with a mechanism similar to EDTA-dependent platelet clumping. A recent study compared the incidence of platelet-monocyte complexes and platelet-neutrophil complexes in peripheral blood (collected with sodium citrate as anticoagulant) from patients with Behcet's disease with and without a history of major vascular involvement. There was an increased incidence of platelet-neutrophil complexes in patients who had major vascular involvement compared to patients without such a history. Thus, platelet satellitism may be more common in patients with this condition.

Case with Error

A 15-year-old female with a history of menorrhagia, renal insufficiency, and hearing loss was referred to a hematologist for management of thrombocytopenia and anemia. Her pediatrician had been treating her for presumptive ITP with intravenous immunoglobulin and steroids, but there was little improvement in the bleeding. CBC data were as follows:

	Result	**Reference Range**
WBC	$8.7 \times 10^3/\mu L$	$3.9-10.7 \times 10^3/\mu L$
Hgb	12.1 g/dL	11.8−16.0 g/dL
Platelets	$15 \times 10^3/\mu L$	$135-371 \times 10^3/\mu L$
Mean platelet volume	14.9 fL	9.3−12.8 fL
Immature platelet fraction	5.4%	0.9%−7.3%

The hematologist recommended splenectomy for symptomatic relief of refractory ITP.

Explanation and Consequences

In this case, the hematologist did not appreciate several clues that the patient's thrombocytopenia might not be due to ITP. While the mean platelet volume (MPV) was elevated, as is typical in ITP, the immature platelet fraction (IPF) was normal. This value is almost invariably high in ITP. Also, the constellation of symptoms of renal insufficiency and hearing loss in conjunction with uniformly large platelets (macrothrombocytopenia) were suggestive of a congenital disease.

The patient's parents wanted a second opinion before consenting to surgery. They visited a second hematologist, who reviewed the peripheral blood smear and noted that the platelets were uniformly large. From the patient's medical history, she suspected a nonmuscle myosin heavy chain 9 (MYH9)-related platelet disorder. An immunofluorescence test was ordered that was positive for protein aggregates within neutrophils. The splenectomy was averted, and the patient's bleeding was treated with platelet transfusion and desmopressin therapy.

MYH9-related disorders are caused by mutations in the *MYH9* gene located on chromosome 22q12-13. All of these syndromes exhibit thrombocytopenia and macrothrombocytopenia. Depending on the specific type of the disease, they may also exhibit hearing loss, nephritis, cataracts, and leukocyte inclusion bodies. A major risk to patients with MYH9-related disorders is misdiagnosis of ITP with resultant inappropriate immunosuppressive therapy and possible splenectomy. Key findings that suggest a MYH9-related disorder are persistent thrombocytopenia unresponsive to conventional ITP therapy and an MPV >12 fL with uniformly large platelets. By contrast, platelets in ITP generally exhibit a gradation of size, with younger large platelets as well as more mature smaller platelets. A family history of thrombocytopenia or bleeding, and a history of cataracts, hearing loss, or renal disease are also suggestive of MYH9-related disorders. Some of these disorders have inclusions in granulocytes that are visible on the Wright-stained peripheral blood smear, as in May-Hegglin anomaly. In others, these inclusions are detectable only by immunofluorescence staining.

Case with Error

A 24-year-old female presents to her internist complaining of gum bleeding and easy bruising. She has a history of neuroblastoma that was treated during childhood, but has been in remission ever since. She has no other signs or symptoms. CBC results are as follows:

	Result	**Reference Range**
WBC	$5.6 \times 10^3/\mu L$	$3.9 - 10.7 \times 10^3/\mu L$
Hgb	14.1 g/dL	11.8 − 16.0 g/dL
Platelets	$17 \times 10^3/\mu L$	$135 - 371 \times 10^3/\mu L$

Understanding the patient's history, the internist is concerned that the thrombocytopenia could indicate relapse of neuroblastoma in the marrow or even secondary myelodysplastic syndrome due to prior exposure to chemotherapy. The patient was referred for platelet transfusion and bone marrow biopsy. The bone marrow was normocellular with trilineage hematopoiesis and a moderate increase in megakaryocytes with a range of morphologies, including some small megakaryocytes with monolobate nuclei. There was no evidence for recurrent neuroblastoma.

Explanation and Consequences

As with any cytopenia, thrombocytopenia can be caused by decreased production, as would be seen in marrow infiltration by tumor or myelodysplastic syndrome. It could also be caused by a peripheral destructive process, such as ITP. These alternatives cannot be distinguished by platelet count alone. However, in this case, the physicians failed to utilize another important tool, the IPF.

The IPF is a measure of platelet immaturity that involves the binding of a fluorescent dye that recognizes ribonucleic acid (RNA). The amount of RNA in the platelet cytoplasm positively corresponds with its immaturity. The normal range for the IPF is 0.9% − 7.0%, and it is typically increased with bone marrow stimulation due to peripheral platelet destruction. In contrast, the IPF is often normal or low in thrombocytopenia due to decreased production.

After reading the bone marrow results, the consulting hematologists recognized the possibility of ITP. An IPF was ordered, and the results were high, at 24%. Based on these findings, the patient was diagnosed with ITP and treated appropriately. However, the initial error delayed this diagnosis and resulted in an invasive and expensive biopsy procedure.

STANDARDS OF CARE

▨ Any new finding of thrombocytopenia should be evaluated by review of the peripheral blood smear. This will help rule out various artifacts, including platelet clumping and platelet satellitosis, which falsely reduce platelet counts produced by automated hematology analyzers. Review of the blood smear will also alert the physician to the presence of large platelets.

▨ Platelet indices, including MPV and the IPF, should be used in conjunction with the platelet count to help determine whether thrombocytopenia is related to production defects or peripheral destruction. It can also help distinguish ITP from less common congenital disorders.

▨ Patients with macrothrombocytopenia that shows uniformity in platelet size should be evaluated with a thorough personal and family history to evaluate for the possibility of a MYH9-related platelet disorder.

RECOMMENDED READING

Althaus K, Greinacher A. MYH-9-related platelet disorders: strategies for management and diagnosis. *Transfus Med Hemother.* 2010;37:260–267.

Pamuk GE, Pamuk ON, Orum H, Demir M, Turgut B, Cakir N. Might platelet-leucocyte complexes be playing a role in major vascular involvement of Behcet's disease? A comparative study. *Blood Coagul Fibrinolysis.* 2010;21:113–117.

Zandecki M, Genevieve F, Gerard J, Godon A. Spurious counts and spurious results on haematology analyzers: a review. Part I: platelets. *Int J Lab Hematol.* 2007;29:4–20.

ERRORS IN THE EVALUATION OF THROMBOCYTOSIS

OVERVIEW

▶ Thrombocytosis may be the first sign of a myeloproliferative disease, such as essential thrombocythemia or primary myelofibrosis, in an as yet asymptomatic patient. However, platelet counts can be elevated in many reactive conditions, including infection, trauma, surgery, and iron deficiency, among others. In addition, platelet counts can be incorrectly presumed to be elevated when a source of small interfering fragments approximately the size of a platelet is present in the blood. Thus, all other causes of thrombocytosis must be ruled out prior to making a diagnosis of myeloproliferative disease.

Case with Error Averted

A 54-year-old male is brought to a trauma center after being pulled from a burning car, with thermal injuries over 90% of his body. As part of his emergency care, a complete blood count (CBC) is ordered, which shows the following results:

	Result	**Reference Range**
WBC	$33.5 \times 10^3/\mu L$	$3.9-10.7 \times 10^3/\mu L$
Hgb	8.5 g/dL	11.8−16.0 g/dL
Platelets	$728 \times 10^3/\mu L$	$135-371 \times 10^3/\mu L$
RBC	$3.0 \times 10^6/\mu l$	$4.0-6.0 \times 10^6/\mu L$
MCV	86 fL	81−98 fL
RDW	23.3%	11.1%−14.3%

Once the patient is stabilized, the trauma team consults hematology to evaluate the high platelet count. They want to know if there needs to be concern for a previously undetected hematologic disorder. The consultant hematologist looks at a peripheral blood smear and notes marked anisopoikilocytosis of the erythrocytes, including numerous microspherocytes and tiny RBC fragments, smaller than the usual schistocytes. They reassure the trauma physicians that there is no concern for a hematologic disorder. Repeat CBC after several days of hospitalization showed a normal platelet count.

Explanation and Consequences

These erythrocyte changes are typical of thermal injury and usually only occur when a significant percentage of the body is burned. The intense heat damages regions of the submembrane spectrin meshwork, causing membrane blebbing and resealing, which results in the formation of small erythrocyte fragments. These fragments can be spuriously counted as platelets by automated hematology analyzers that detect platelets using size distributions only. Thus, the reported platelet count is much higher than the actual platelet count, and this falsely high value raised concern for myeloproliferative disease.

In this case, the hematologist appropriately looked at a peripheral blood smear and recognized the hallmarks of thermal injury, including the presence of numerous small erythrocyte fragments. She correctly concluded that these were likely responsible for the high platelet count and decided to wait for the results of subsequent CBCs before acting further.

This error will be prevented by new hematology analyzers that detect platelets using a combination of size and either fluorescent dyes that recognize DNA and RNA or by antibodies against platelet-specific antigens. These techniques can effectively distinguish between erythrocyte fragments and genuine platelets.

Case with Error

A 48-year-old man complains to his physician about a lack of energy at a regular check-up. On examination, the physician notes conjunctival pallor and mild tachycardia. CBC results are as follows:

	Result	**Reference Range**
WBC	$4.8 \times 10^3/\mu L$	$3.9-10.7 \times 10^3/\mu L$
Hgb	11.1 g/dL	11.8−16.0 g/dL
Platelets	$792 \times 10^3/\mu L$	$135-371 \times 10^3/\mu L$
RBC	$3.5 \times 10^6/\mu L$	$4.0-6.0 \times 10^6/\mu L$
MCV	76 fL	81−98 fL
RDW	16.4%	11.1%−14.3%

The physician notes microcytic anemia and appropriately follows up with iron studies, which indicate iron deficiency. He prescribes oral iron supplements, but remains concerned about the patient's thrombocytosis. Consequently, the physician refers the patient to a hematologist for a bone marrow biopsy to rule out a myeloproliferative neoplasm.

Explanation and Consequences

In this case the physician did not recognize that thrombocytosis can be caused by iron deficiency. In fact, some have referred to the platelet count as a "poor man's iron study." This occurs because iron is an inhibitor of thrombopoiesis; thus, decreased iron storage stimulates platelet production. Failure to recognize this correlation resulted in an inappropriate differential diagnosis and an unnecessary referral.

The hematologist noted the patient's history of iron deficiency and canceled the bone marrow biopsy. Instead, he followed up with a CBC after the patient had been on oral iron therapy for 3 months, at which point the platelet count had decreased to $335 \times 10^3/\mu L$, which is within the normal range.

Case with Error

A 42-year-old female presents to the emergency department after 4 days of progressive fatigue, nausea, and headache. She has a history of acute myeloid leukemia diagnosed 6 months earlier. She had been in complete remission after chemotherapy. On exam she was not short of breath and did not have any bleeding, petechiae, or bruises. Her CBC was as follows:

	Result	**Reference Range**
WBC	$133 \times 10^3/\mu L$	$3.9-10.7 \times 10^3/\mu L$
Hgb	7.7 g/dL	11.8−16.0 g/dL
Platelets	$402 \times 10^3/\mu L$	$135-371 \times 10^3/\mu L$

Review of the peripheral blood smear reveals numerous blasts and what look like adequate numbers of platelets. The patient is diagnosed with relapsed leukemia and admitted for treatment. A surgeon is asked to place a central line for chemotherapy administration. He checks the platelet count, and finding it adequate, he proceeds to place the line. However, the procedure is complicated by excessive and prolonged bleeding, and the patient develops a large hematoma at the site.

Explanation and Consequences

In this case, the platelet count was spuriously elevated because of tumor lysis, a syndrome of tumor cell breakdown that can occur spontaneously in individuals with high tumor burden or as a result of chemotherapy. In this context, the degrading blasts may break into small fragments that appear to be platelets, both to automated analyzers and visually on the blood smear.

The patient outcome prompted a second review of the blood smear. A supervising technologist recognized the leukocyte fragments and was able to distinguish them from platelets due to a more basophilic color and the presence of nuclear material in some fragments. She estimated the actual platelet count at $7 \times 10^3/\mu L$. If this had been reported initially, the patient would have received a platelet transfusion prior to the procedure that may have prevented the bleeding complications.

In this case, there were two clues that, if recognized, could have prevented this error. First, the hematology analyzer flagged the specimen for "abnormal platelet distribution," indicating that the platelet size distribution was abnormal. Second, review of a recent CBC from an outside clinic showed that the patient's platelet count was $42 \times 10^3/\mu L$ several days prior to presentation. It would have been unusual for her platelet count to increase this significantly in a few days, especially in the context of relapsing leukemia. If the clinicians had recognized this anomaly, they may have raised suspicions that the high "platelet count" was an artifact.

Case with Error

A 45-year-old female undergoes a splenectomy to treat long-standing autoimmune hemolytic anemia. At a 1-month follow-up appointment, CBC values are as follows:

	Result	**Reference Range**
WBC	$8.3 \times 10^3/\mu L$	$3.9 - 10.7 \times 10^3/\mu L$
Hgb	13.0 g/dL	$11.8 - 16.0$ g/dL
Platelets	$1,146 \times 10^3/\mu L$	$135 - 371 \times 10^3/\mu L$

The surgeon notes resolution of the patient's anemia, but is concerned about the markedly elevated platelet count. He refers the patient to a hematologist for a bone marrow biopsy to rule out a myeloproliferative process.

Explanation and Consequences

The surgeon mistakenly concluded that the high platelet count may be indicative of a hematologic disorder. However, he did not realize that thrombocytosis is a common consequence of splenectomy, occurring in 75%–80% of patients. In general, the platelet count increases in the first few weeks after surgery and can reach levels in excess of $1,000 \times 10^3/\mu L$ before gradually returning to normal. However, the rate of normalization is variable and may extend to months, or even years, after the procedure.

This error led to an inappropriate referral and could have resulted in an unnecessary procedure. However, the hematologist recognized that thrombocytosis is common in this clinical setting. In addition, she reviewed the peripheral smear, and found that the erythrocytes exhibited anisopoikilocytosis, basophilic stippling, and Howell-Jolly bodies, which are also sequelae of a splenectomy. Thus, the bone marrow biopsy was canceled, and the patient was reassured.

STANDARDS OF CARE

▨ A peripheral blood smear should be reviewed for all patients with a new diagnosis of thrombocytosis in order to confirm that the platelet count is likely to be correct, and to exclude possible spurious causes of high platelet count.

▨ Thrombocytosis in the presence of iron deficiency should be considered reactive. Additional evaluation for thrombocytosis should not be performed unless the platelet count does not normalize with iron therapy.

▨ Other causes of reactive thrombocytosis should be excluded before referring a patient for evaluation of possible myeloproliferative disease.

▨ An "abnormal platelet distribution" flag from a hematology analyzer or a rapid, significant change in platelet count should trigger a manual smear review and platelet count estimate.

▨ In situations where tumor lysis is a possibility, leukocyte fragments should be excluded as a possible cause of an inaccurate platelet count before any procedures are performed.

RECOMMENDED READING

Glassy EF, ed. *Color Atlas of Hematology: An Illustrated Field Guide Based on Proficiency Testing*. Northfield, IL: CAP Press; 1998.

Zandecki M, Genevieve F, Gerard J, Godon A. Spurious counts and spurious results on haematology analyzers: a review. Part I: platelets. *Int J Lab Hematol*. 2007;29:4–20.

II

IMMUNOLOGY

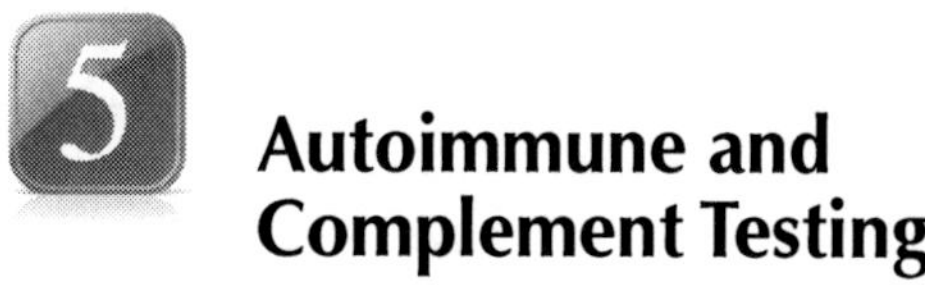

Autoimmune and Complement Testing

ERRORS IN THE INTERPRETATION OF ANTINUCLEAR ANTIBODY TESTS

OVERVIEW

Antinuclear antibodies (ANAs) are autoantibodies directed against antigens found in the nucleus of many cells. These antigens include double-stranded DNA (dsDNA), centromere proteins, histones, topoisomerases, and constituents of the small nuclear ribonucleoproteins (snRNPs), among others. ANAs are most often detected in patients with autoimmune collagen vascular diseases, including systemic lupus erythematosus (SLE), systemic sclerosis, Sjögren's syndrome, inflammatory myopathies, and mixed connective tissue disease, although they can be seen to some degree in other disorders and occasional healthy patients. They are most commonly detected by indirect fluorescence assay (IFA) using standardized cultured human cells, such as Hep-2 cells. When positive, the fluorescence appears as distinct patterns in the interphase and mitotic cells, and these patterns correlate with specific nuclear antigens and specific collagen vascular diseases. The most common patterns are smooth/homogeneous, speckled, centromeric, and nucleolar, although some laboratories recognize additional patterns. Positive results are typically reported with the pattern and a titer, which is the highest dilution of serum at which fluorescence is detected.

Positive ANAs are often followed by testing for extractable nuclear antigens (ENAs), which represent the specific antigens targeted by ANAs. Many ENAs have been described, but most laboratories test for common subsets that have particular disease associations, some of which are listed in the table on the next page. ENA testing is typically performed using an enzyme immunoassay (EIA) platform.

Extractable Nuclear Antigens (ENAs)

ENA Name	Antigen Target	ANA Pattern	Disease Association
Anti-dsDNA	Native DNA	Smooth/homogeneous	SLE
Anti-histone	Histones	Smooth/homogeneous	SLE (especially drug-induced)
Anti-Sm	Ribonucleoprotein	Speckled or smooth	SLE
Anti-Ro (SS-A)	Ribonucleoprotein	Speckled	Sjögren syndrome or SLE
Anti-La (SS-B)	Ribonucleoprotein	Speckled	Sjögren syndrome or SLE
Anti-U1-RNP	Ribonucleoprotein	Speckled	Mixed connective tissue disease
Anti-Scl-70	DNA topoisomerase	Speckled or nucleolar	Systemic sclerosis
Anti-centromere	Centromere proteins	Centromeric	Limited scleroderma

Case with Error

A 42-year-old man presents to his primary care physician complaining of worsening joint pain and fatigue over a period of 2–3 months. The pain is worst in both knees and in the shoulder joints and seems to be unrelated to exertion. He also complains of an itchy rash on his chest that has developed over the same time period. Review of symptoms is otherwise negative. Physical examination is unremarkable, except for an eczematous rash on the chest. His ANA is positive with a speckled pattern and a titer of 1:80. Laboratory studies including complete blood count (CBC), C-reactive protein (CRP), erythrocyte sedimentation rate, and complement levels are normal. A presumptive diagnosis of

SLE is made, glucocorticoid therapy is initiated, and the patient is referred to a rheumatologist.

Explanation and Consequences

In this case, the physician overinterpreted the ANA result to make a diagnosis of SLE, despite the fact that the clinical signs and symptoms did not meet criteria for the diagnosis. Complaints of fatigue and arthralgia are common in primary care. In conjunction with a dermatologic finding, as found in this patient, suspicion is often raised for one of several autoimmune diseases. It is common practice to screen for autoimmune diseases using the ANA test. However, while quite sensitive for the diagnosis of collagen vascular diseases, the test may be positive in patients with many other conditions. The ANA is frequently positive (up to 50%) in patients with rheumatologic disorders other than collagen vascular disease, in patients with infectious diseases, and in patients with malignancies. In fact, 20%–30% of otherwise healthy, asymptomatic patients have a positive ANA at a titer of 1:40. This problem can be ameliorated somewhat by raising the threshold titer for a positive test. However, up to 5% of healthy patients may have an ANA titer of 1:160, and raising the threshold titer significantly decreases sensitivity for detecting collagen vascular disorders.

An unfortunate consequence of the low specificity of the ANA test is a decrease in positive predictive value, which is the proportion of patients with a positive test that have the disease. In a typical screening population, the majority of patients with a positive ANA do not actually have a collagen vascular disease. Thus, using the ANA for a general screening test in patients with nonspecific complaints is not often diagnostically informative and can be misleading. The positive predictive value can be significantly improved by restricting use of the ANA test to patients with a higher pretest probability of collagen vascular disease.

The American College of Rheumatology publishes specific criteria for the diagnosis of rheumatologic disorders, including the collagen vascular disorders. For example, to diagnose SLE a patient must have 4 of the following 11 signs and symptoms: malar rash, discoid rash, photosensitivity, oral ulcers, arthritis, serositis, renal disease, neurologic disorder, hematologic disorder, immunologic disorder, and a positive ANA result. The patient described in the case above met only two or three of these criteria, depending on the interpretation of the rash. Thus, a diagnosis of SLE is not appropriate in this case, and glucocorticoid therapy should not have been initiated in the absence of another rheumatologic disorder that is treated with glucocorticoids. Inappropriate therapy could have been avoided by not ordering the ANA test in this patient with a low pretest probability of collagen vascular disease.

Case with Error

A 64-year-old man presents to a pulmonary clinic with a 5-year history of worsening respiratory symptoms, including dry cough and dyspnea on exertion. Review of systems is otherwise negative, with no history of arthralgia or myalgia, rash or other dermatopathology, Raynaud's phenomenon, and other constitutional symptoms. He has a history of hypertension, hyperlipidemia, and coronary artery disease with a myocardial infarction 10 years prior to this presentation. Chest x-ray shows interstitial infiltrates bilaterally, and pulmonary function tests are consistent with restrictive pulmonary disease. The pulmonologist strongly suspects idiopathic pulmonary fibrosis. However, a panel of rheumatologic tests, including ANA and a complete ENA panel, are ordered to rule out an underlying autoimmune disease, such as systemic sclerosis. The ANA is negative. However, the anti-dsDNA test is positive (179 IU/mL; normal <25 IU/mL). Concerned for a collagen vascular disease, the patient was referred to a rheumatologist for treatment.

Explanation and Consequences

In this case, the physician inappropriately interpreted a positive anti-dsDNA as being indicative of autoimmune disease in the absence of a positive ANA and appropriate signs and symptoms. Anti-dsDNA antibodies are recognized as a type of antinuclear antibodies that have particularly high prevalence in patients with SLE (40%–60%). Traditionally, they have been assayed by an indirect IFA using the protist *Crithidia luciliae* as a substrate. Similar to the ANA test, the results are expressed as a titer. This assay, used specifically to detect anti-dsDNA antibodies, detects high-affinity antibodies and is very specific for SLE. In fact, it is uncommon to see positive results in healthy patients or in those with collagen vascular diseases other than SLE.

However, because this test methodology is more costly and labor intensive, many laboratories have transitioned to a different method (EIA) for anti-dsDNA testing. This method involves the use of recombinant DNA or DNA purified from an animal source. This assay is more sensitive, but less specific for SLE than the IFA method, perhaps due to its propensity to detect clinically insignificant low-affinity antibodies. This is likely what happened in the case described above, generating a false-positive result.

This outcome could have been avoided by more judicious use of ENA testing. The patient's symptoms in this case were not consistent with SLE, the disorder in which anti-dsDNA antibodies are most commonly seen. Thus, the pretest probability of a true-positive result was very low. Consensus guidelines recommend that tests for specific ENAs should be restricted to patients who have a positive ANA. Despite this, some clinicians order ENAs at the same time as the ANA, so that patients will not need to come in for a second blood draw should the ANA return positive. To avoid this practice, many laboratories offer reflex testing of ENAs based on algorithmic protocols that stop ENA testing if the ANA test is negative. In at least one study, this resulted in lower ENA utilization, and a higher fraction of positive ENA tests, suggesting that there is an increased positive predictive value for the ENA using this approach.

STANDARDS OF CARE

▓ ANA testing should be performed only in patients for whom there is a high clinical suspicion of collagen vascular disease based on defined diagnostic guidelines. It should not be used as a general screening test. This approach will increase positive predictive values and decrease false-positive results.

▓ Even when ordered appropriately, ANA results must be interpreted in the proper clinical context. Diagnosis of collagen vascular disease should not be based on ANA testing alone, but in concert

with clinical findings and supportive radiographic and laboratory testing.
■ Testing for specific ENAs should be restricted to patients known to have a positive ANA test.

RECOMMENDED READING

Kavanaugh A, Tomar R, Reveille J, Solomon DH, Homburger HA. Guidelines for clinical use of the antinuclear antibody test and tests for specific autoantibodies to nuclear antigens. *Arch Pathol Lab Med.* 2000;124:71–81.

Meroni PL, Schur PH. ANA screening: an old test with new recommendations. *Ann Rheum Dis.* 2010;69:1420–1422.

Satoh M, Vazques-Del Mercado M, Chan EK. Clinical interpretation of antinuclear antibody tests in systemic rheumatic diseases. *Mod Rheumatol.* 2009;19:219–228.

Wahed A, Risin S. Issues with Immunology and Serology Testing. In: Dasgupta A, Sepulveda JL, eds. *Accurate Results in the Clinical Laboratory: A Guide to Error Detection and Correction.* Amsterdam, Netherlands: Elsevier; 2013:295–304.

ERRORS IN THE INTERPRETATION OF THE RHEUMATOID FACTOR TEST

OVERVIEW

▶ Rheumatoid factor (RF) is often elevated in the plasma or serum of patients with rheumatoid arthritis (RA) and has long been used as a tool in the diagnosis of this disease. However, the RF test is not specific. It can be elevated in a number of other conditions and occasionally in healthy patients. Thus, it is important to interpret RF results in clinical context and to rule out other associated diagnoses before making a diagnosis of RA.

Case with Error

A 59-year-old man presents to his primary care physician complaining of nonspecific systemic symptoms, the most prominent of which are low-grade fever and joint pain. Physical examination reveals reddish raised nodules over several knuckles. Laboratory tests reveal a slightly elevated white blood cell (WBC) count at $13.4 \times 10^3/\mu L$, with a normal WBC differential. The erythrocyte sedimentation rate (ESR) and C-reactive protein (CRP) are elevated. As the differential diagnosis includes RA, an RF test is performed, which is positive. The physician diagnoses the patient with RA and refers him to a rheumatologist.

The rheumatologist feels that the history and physical examination findings, while suspicious, are not entirely typical of RA. Additionally, he notes a mild cardiac murmur, most consistent with mitral regurgitation. Serial blood cultures are positive for *Staphylococcus aureus* and mitral regurgitation is confirmed by echocardiogram. A diagnosis of infective endocarditis is made and antibiotic therapy is initiated.

Explanation and Consequences

In this case, the primary care physician used a positive RF as definitive evidence for the diagnosis of RA, without recognizing its lack of specificity for RA and investigating other possible diagnoses that could have overlapping symptoms with RA and similar laboratory results. He also did not confirm the diagnosis of RA with a more specific test.

RA is a systemic autoimmune disease, the hallmark of which is joint inflammation, leading to pain, swelling, and stiffness, although other organs are frequently affected. As in this case, the diagnosis of RA can be challenging, especially in the early stages. In addition to joint pain, there are often nonspecific constitutional symptoms, including fever, fatigue, and malaise, that overlap with a number of other conditions. Serologic tests and assays for generalized inflammation, such as ESR and CRP, thus play an important role in the evaluation of a patient for RA.

RF is an autoantibody with specificity for the Fc portion of immunoglobulin G (IgG). It was first associated with RA in the 1940s and, therefore, has long been used as a diagnostic test for this disorder. Today, it remains part of the most recent RA classification criteria endorsed by the American College of Rheumatology (ACR). However, the interpretation of a positive RF test is challenging. It is not very sensitive, as up to 30% of RA patients are negative, especially in the early stages of the disease when the diagnosis is most difficult. A positive test is not specific for RA, as RF is positive in a number of other autoimmune and inflammatory conditions. In fact, a positive RF is a frequent finding in most collagen vascular diseases, particularly Sjögren syndrome. It is detected in many chronic infections, including up to half of patients with infectious endocarditis or viral hepatitis. RF can also be positive in patients with pulmonary diseases, such as sarcoidosis and interstitial fibrosis, other autoimmune diseases, and cancer. Finally, a small percentage of otherwise healthy individuals are also positive for RF, and this frequency increases with age.

Due to these limitations, overreliance on RF for the diagnosis of RA can lead to a misdiagnosis. In the case described above, the patient had infective endocarditis, the symptoms of which are similarly nonspecific. These include low-grade fever, fatigue, musculoskeletal pain, and malaise. The characteristic subcutaneous nodules of endocarditis, termed Osler's nodes, can be mistaken for the rheumatoid nodules seen in RA. Systemic inflammation, which is associated with elevated ESR and CRP values, is a common feature of both diseases. Endocarditis is a serious disease, and the error resulted in a delay in appropriate treatment that had significant adverse consequences in this case.

Additional serologic tests have been developed to improve the accuracy of the diagnosis of RA. Anticitrullinated peptide antibody (ACPA) tests, such as anticyclic citrullinated peptide (CCP), are at least as sensitive (70%–78%) and are more specific (88%–96%) than the RF test. ACPA tests are listed as alternative assays to the RF test, with equal weight in the ACR diagnostic criteria. Consequently, some institutions and practitioners have switched entirely from RF to anti-CCP testing. Anti-CCP was eventually shown to be negative in the case described above.

Even with these improvements, careful history and physical examination and good clinical judgment are generally superior to serologic testing in the diagnosis of RA, especially when the pretest probability is low or high. The value of tests for RA is in intermediate probability scenarios, when the history and physical findings are inconclusive.

STANDARDS OF CARE

▨ Serologic testing, whether using RF or anti-CCP, should be restricted to cases with intermediate diagnostic probability by history and physical examination.

▨ The RF test should not be relied upon as the sole serologic test in the diagnosis of RA. ACPA tests, such as anti-CCP, which are more specific, should be utilized with or instead of RF.

▨ Positive RF tests should be interpreted carefully, as positive results are common in patients with other diseases, many of which have clinical features that significantly overlap with those of RA. Thus, these other disorders should be considered in the differential diagnosis until ruled out.

RECOMMENDED READING

Aletaha D, Neogi T, Silman AJ, et al. 2010. Rheumatoid arthritis classification criteria: an American College of Rheumatology/European League Against Rheumatism collaborative initiative. *Arthritis Rheum.* 2010;62:2569–2581.

Beck CE, Hall M. Rheumatoid factor and anti-CCP autoantibodies in rheumatoid arthritis: a review. *Clin Lab Sci.* 2008;21:15–18.

ERRORS IN THE INTERPRETATION OF ANTINEUTROPHIL CYTOPLASMIC ANTIBODY TESTS

OVERVIEW

Antineutrophil cytoplasmic antibodies (ANCA) are auto-antibodies most commonly associated with a group of severe systemic vasculitis syndromes, including Wegener's granulomatosis, Churg-Strauss syndrome, and microscopic polyangiitis, collectively known as ANCA-associated vasculitides (AAVs). The ANCA test is performed by an indirect immunofluorescence test in which patient serum is exposed to human neutrophils. In a positive test, application of a secondary fluorescently tagged antihuman IgG antibody reveals cytoplasmic positivity on formalin-fixed neutrophils. In ethanol-fixed neutrophils, one of two distinct patterns will emerge. Using this methodology, persistent cytoplasmic positivity is referred to as c-ANCA, while a perinuclear pattern is called p-ANCA. Autoantibodies against a number of different antigens can be responsible for ANCAs. However, the most common are myeloperoxidase (MPO) in p-ANCA and proteinase 3 (PR3) in c-ANCA, both of which are detected by enzyme immunoassay (EIA). Vasculitides are serious diseases with potentially high morbidity and mortality, and, thus, early definitive diagnosis is critical to effective therapy. However, these serologic tests can be positive in other, less severe nonvasculitic disorders and after exposure to certain drugs, and, thus, can be misdiagnosed as AAVs.

Case with Error

A 33-year-old woman presents to her physician complaining of a recent history of fatigue, malaise, sore joints and muscles, and skin rashes. Routine laboratory testing is significant for mild normocytic anemia and increased serum creatinine. Urinalysis shows hematuria and proteinuria, raising concern for acute renal failure. Upon questioning, the patient indicates that she had been healthy until 4 months earlier, when she was diagnosed with Graves' disease, for which she was treated with propylthiouracil (PTU). As part of the evaluation for renal failure, autoimmune serologies are performed, showing a positive ANCA test with a perinuclear pattern (p-ANCA). EIA is positive for anti-MPO. She is referred to a rheumatologist with a diagnosis of microscopic polyangiitis and immunosuppressant therapy is initiated, which includes prednisone and cyclosporine.

Explanation and Consequences

In this case, the physician did not understand that the clinical and laboratory features of AAVs could also be seen in drug-induced vasculitis. Drug-induced vasculitis presents with nonspecific constitutional symptoms, including fever, malaise, arthralgia, myalgia, and weight loss. Anemia and skin rashes are also common. Specific organ system involvement is most common in the kidneys, where glomerulonephritis with hematuria, proteinuria, and rising creatinine is often observed. Importantly, the ANCA test is positive in drug-induced vasculitis and typically has a perinuclear (p-ANCA) pattern on ethanol-fixed neutrophils. Associated anti-MPO antibodies are most common, although autoantibodies to other antigens can also be present.

A number of drugs are associated with drug-induced vasculitis. The most common of these are antithyroid drugs, such as PTU, which are used to treat hyperthyroidism. Other drugs implicated include hydralazine, sulfasalazine, D-penicillamine, and minocycline. Recent case reports have also associated anti-TNF-α drugs, such as infliximab, with drug-induced vasculitis.

The primary features distinguishing drug-induced vasculitides from systemic AAVs are a milder clinical course and clear association with drug administration. Importantly, withdrawal of the drug often results in reversal of both clinical and serologic manifestations of the disease, especially early in the disease course, and relapses can be prevented by future avoidance of the implicated drug. In more severe cases of drug-induced vasculitis, immunosuppressant therapy may be required. However, the required course of therapy is often shorter and long-term maintenance is not generally required for lasting remission. Thus, in this case, proper diagnosis of drug-induced vasculitis would have prompted cessation of PTU, and may have prevented the use of immunosuppressants with their potential complications.

Case with Error

A 36-year-old male presents to an otolaryngology clinic complaining of a several-month history of sinonasal congestion, pain, and epistaxis that is not relieved by decongestants or antibiotics. Examination reveals edema and a nasal septal perforation. The nasal epithelium is biopsied and shows extensive acute and chronic inflammation, without discernable granulomas. Cultures of the nasal epithelium are positive for *Staphylococcus aureus.* Serologic testing is significant for a positive c-ANCA test with a titer >1:160 that is specific for PR-3 on EIA. A diagnosis of Wegener's granulomatosis (also known as granulomatosis with polyangiitis, or GPA) is made, and immunosuppressant therapy is initiated.

Explanation and Consequences

As in the prior case, the physician did not properly interpret the ANCA test in clinical context. The presenting features of Wegener's granulomatosis often include sinonasal symptoms, and it can cause destruction of bone and cartilage, leading to nasal septal or palatal defects. However, these clinical features overlap with other diseases, especially early in the disease course. Among the similar disorders is cocaine-induced midline destructive lesion (CIMDL). This is a disease of chronic cocaine abusers in which the primary route of cocaine administration is nasal inhalation. These patients also experience chronic sinonasal inflammation with associated congestion and pain. Similar to Wegener's granulomatosis, they develop destructive osteo-cartilaginous lesions, including nasal septal and palatal defects. In this case, a urine drug screen performed later was positive for cocaine in this patient, and he admitted almost daily use.

Importantly, patients with CIMDL may have positive ANCA serologies, typically with c-ANCA/PR3 specificity, although p-ANCA has also been reported. In addition to anti-PR3, patients with CIMDL often have antihuman neutrophil elastase (anti-HNE) antibodies, which are seen in drug-induced vasculitis, but not in Wegener's granulomatosis. Thus, this antibody may help rule out Wegener's granulomatosis, although it is typically available only in highly specialized clinical laboratories.

Biopsies of nasal mucosa in Wegener's granulomatosis typically show acute vascular inflammation with associated granulomas. However, small biopsies may not be adequate to see all of these features. Indeed, nearly half of biopsies are insufficient to make the diagnosis. Therefore, the absence of clear vasculitis and granulomas in the biopsy of this case does not rule out the disease.

Differentiation of CIMDL from Wegener's granulomatosis is critical, as the treatments are drastically different. Unlike Wegener's granulomatosis, immunosuppression does not play a role in the therapy of CIMDL. Rather, cessation of cocaine use coupled with surgical repair of destructive lesions is the most appropriate response. Recognition of the overlapping clinical and laboratory features of these disorders could have prevented initiation of immunosuppressant therapy, with its accompanying side effects.

Case with Error

A 23-year-old male presents with a 2-week history of watery diarrhea. He reports occasional blood-tinged stools. The episodes of diarrhea are associated with cramping abdominal pain and low-grade fever. He has decreased appetite and has lost 12 pounds since the onset of symptoms. He says that he had a similar episode about a year earlier that spontaneously resolved. His physician expresses concern for inflammatory bowel disease (IBD) and orders a series of tests for autoimmunity. Among these, ANCA testing is positive with a c-ANCA pattern. EIA tests are positive for anti-PR3 and negative for anti-MPO. Colonoscopy is performed and biopsies show ulceration with acute inflammation and crypt abscesses. A diagnosis of Crohn's disease (CD) is made and immunosuppressive therapy is initiated with no relief of symptoms.

Explanation and Consequences

As in the prior cases, the error is a failure to recognize the relatively low specificity of the ANCA test and to consider other possible disorders in the differential diagnosis. In this case, when immune suppression failed to ameliorate the patient's symptoms, additional studies were performed, including stool cultures and an ova and parasite examination. These revealed increased fecal leukocytes and *Entamoeba histolytica* infection.

IBDs are autoimmune inflammatory disorders of the gastrointestinal tract, and include CD and ulcerative colitis (UC). Although each of these diagnoses has some distinctive clinical features, both usually present with some combination of abdominal pain, cramping, diarrhea, rectal bleeding, and weight loss. Additionally, ANCA testing can be positive in both forms of IBD. Approximately 10%–20% of patients with CD and 40%–80% of patients with UC have positive ANCA serologies, usually with an atypical pattern.

While a positive ANCA test can be supportive of a diagnosis of IBD, care should be taken to rule out infectious etiologies. Amebic dysentery, caused by infection with *E. histolytica*, presents with clinical symptoms that are very similar to those of IBD. In addition, gross findings on colonoscopy and the microscopic appearance on biopsy show significant overlap between IBD and amebic dysentery. Serologic findings may also be similar. Approximately 90% of patients with amebiasis carry ANCA antibodies, which are most often cytoplasmic (c-ANCA) with anti-PR3 specificity. This may distinguish amebiasis from IBD, which usually has an atypical ANCA pattern and is negative for both anti-MPO and anti-PR3 tests.

Distinguishing between IBD and amebiasis is crucial, as the immunosuppressant therapy commonly employed in the treatment of IBD may increase severity of amoeba infections. Thus, it is crucial to keep amebic dysentery in the differential diagnosis and not to over-interpret serologic tests, such as the ANCA test.

Case with Error

A 20-year-old male being evaluated for chronic hypertension is found to have renal insufficiency with a decreased glomerular filtration rate. The patient complains of exertional chest pain and fatigue. The remaining review of systems is negative. The patient specifically denies fever, loss of appetite, and weight loss. Physical examination is normal except for moderate hypertension. Urinalysis reveals mild proteinuria with no hematuria. The erythrocyte sedimentation rate and C-reactive protein are normal, as is the complete blood count (CBC). As part of the routine evaluation, ANCA testing is ordered, which is negative. EIA for anti-PR3 is negative, but anti-MPO is mildly elevated at 8.1 units/mL (negative <4, equivocal 4–6, positive >6 EU/mL). The patient is immediately referred to a rheumatologist with a provisional diagnosis of microscopic polyangiitis (MPA).

Explanation and Consequences

In this case, ANCA serologies were ordered as a screening test, even though the patient lacked symptoms and laboratory findings of an AAV. This approach led to a false-positive anti-MPO test and an inappropriate referral, delaying diagnosis and definitive therapy. Fortunately, the rheumatologist recognized the error and ordered a renal biopsy that revealed focal segmental glomerulosclerosis with no evidence of vasculitis.

ANCA testing and the associated EIAs for anti-MPO and PR3 antibodies are adjunctive tests that support a diagnosis of AAV when positive. However, they cannot be relied upon as the sole diagnostic indicator for these diseases. A diagnosis of AAV should be rendered only when there is strong clinical, laboratory, and/or histologic evidence of disease in conjunction with positive serology. In the case described above, the patient presented with renal insufficiency and proteinuria, which can be presenting features of MPA. However, these findings are nonspecific, as they are present in many conditions associated with renal failure. Furthermore, the patient lacked the constitutional signs and symptoms, as well as the laboratory findings that are common in MPA.

The danger in ordering ANCA as a screening test is the risk of generating false-positive results. These occur at some rate in almost every test, but the risk is increased when testing is performed in patients with a low pretest probability of the disease. In this situation, the positive predictive value (PPV), defined as the fraction of patients with a positive test that actually have the disease, is low. Consequently, many, if not most, positive tests are false positives. The

PPV can be increased by restricting testing to patients with a high pretest probability of disease.

Another problem with the serologic findings in this case is that there is a positive anti-MPO EIA, even though the ANCA test (by indirect immunofluorescence) is negative. As indicated in the overview above, a positive anti-MPO test is usually associated with a positive ANCA test with a c-ANCA pattern. Given that the level of MPO is relatively low, these findings are most consistent with a false-positive MPO test and thus do not constitute serologic evidence of an AAV, especially in the absence of appropriate clinical features.

There are exceptions to these rules. Rarely, patients with a bona fide AAV will have a negative ANCA test by indirect immunofluorescence, but a positive EIA for anti-MPO or anti-PR3. However, in these situations, the anti-MPO or anti-PR3 levels are typically much higher than is seen in this case and must be accompanied by a classical clinical syndrome. In fact, a presumptive diagnosis of AAV can be made even with completely negative serologies if the clinical presentation and other histologic and laboratory features are strongly indicative of an AAV.

STANDARDS OF CARE

▓ ANCA tests should be ordered only in the proper clinical context; that is, when there is a high index of suspicion for AAV based on clinical and laboratory findings.

▓ Positive ANCA test results are nonspecific. Other causes of positive ANCA tests include medications, drugs, infections, and other nonvasculitic autoimmune diseases (e.g., inflammatory bowel disease or autoimmune hepatitis). These must be ruled out before a diagnosis of AAV is rendered. This approach will decrease the probability of inappropriate diagnosis and therapy.

▓ Regardless of serologic results, a diagnosis of AAV should not be rendered in the absence of appropriate clinical, laboratory, and/or histologic evidence of disease. This is of particular concern when there is discordance between negative ANCA test results by immunofluorescence and positive anti-MPO or anti-PR3 results by EIA. Conversely, a positive ANCA test result is not required to make a presumptive diagnosis of AAV if the clinical suspicion is high.

RECOMMENDED READING

Bosch X, Guilabert A, Font J. Antineutrophil cytoplasmic antibodies. *Lancet*. 2006;368:404–418.

Csernok E, Lamprecht P, Gross WL. Clinical and immunological features of drug-induced and infection-induced proteinase 3-antineutrophil cytoplasmic antibodies and myeloperoxidase-antineutrophil cytoplasmic antibodies and vasculitis. *Curr Opin Rheumatol*. 2010;22:43–48.

Savige J, Pollock W, Trevisin M. What do antineutrophil cytoplasmic antibodies (ANCA) tell us? *Best Pract Res Clin Rheumatol*. 2005;19:263–276.

ERRORS IN THE INTERPRETATION OF COMPLEMENT TESTING

OVERVIEW

The complement system is a series of blood proteins produced by the liver that act in concert with the innate and adaptive immune systems to clear pathogens. In the process of activations, these proteins act variously to lyse cells, to opsonize organisms for phagocytosis, and to activate the immune system by acting as chemoattractants for leukocytes. In clinical practice, measurement of the complement system is used to diagnose deficiencies in the complement system. Low complement levels can be found in patients with congenital complement deficiencies, and in those with increased formation of immune complexes. These include autoimmune disorders, such as systemic lupus erythematosus (SLE), and renal diseases, especially various types of glomerulonephritis. In these cases, low complement levels are caused by consumption, as immune complexes activate the complement system. For this reason, complement measurement can be used to monitor disease activity.

Common complement measurements include hemolytic complement activity, or CH50, which measures total complement pathway activity by assessing the ability of the patient serum to lyse sheep red blood cells. Antigenic tests for total serum levels of complement factors C3 and C4 are also available.

Case with Error

A 35-year-old woman was diagnosed 7 years ago with SLE. Primary manifestations of her disease were renal insufficiency, arthritis, and dermatitis. However, her disease has been reasonably well controlled with intermittent immunosuppression for occasional flares. Disease activity has been routinely monitored with serum C3 levels, which have been within normal range for years. With her disease stable, she decides to become pregnant. Her pregnancy is uneventful until the third trimester, when she begins to exhibit proteinuria and hypertension. Her C3 level is 104 mg/dL, which is lower than her baseline level of approximately 150 mg/dL, but still within the normal range for the test (88–201 mg/dL). Consequently, this is not considered evidence of a lupus flare, but rather evidence of early preeclampsia, and appropriate therapy for preeclampsia is initiated.

Explanation and Consequences

In this case, the physician did not understand the effect of pregnancy on complement levels and, thus, misdiagnosed a lupus flare as early preeclampsia. While complement levels are an effective way to monitor the disease activity of immune complex-mediated disorders such as SLE, it is important to recognize that complement levels can be modulated by a number of nonimmune complex-related conditions. The effects of these conditions on complement levels and activity must be taken into account when interpreting complement test results.

Complement factors are acute phase proteins and, thus, are increased in inflammatory conditions, such as infections or noninfectious chronic inflammatory disorders. They also increase during pregnancy, particularly in the second and third trimesters. Consequently, the hypocomplementemia associated with immune complex-mediated diseases may not be apparent in these conditions. In pregnancy, C3 levels may be normal in active disease. Thus, it is important to assess the change in C3 levels in serial samples, rather than make conclusions from a single value. In this case, the C3 levels decreased from baseline, suggesting a reactivation of disease, which is a common occurrence in pregnancy. Failure to recognize this led to misdiagnosis of this patient and inappropriate therapy, markedly increasing the risk of poor fetal outcome.

Interpretation of complement tests can also be complicated by conditions that decrease complement levels in the absence of immune complex formation. These include cholesterol embolism (atheroembolism), severe sepsis, thrombotic thrombocytopenic purpura, hemolytic uremic syndrome, acute pancreatitis, malnutrition, and severe liver disease, among others. Several of these conditions have signs or symptoms that overlap with immune complex-mediated diseases. Thus, it is critical to consider these conditions in the differential diagnosis of low complement levels.

STANDARDS OF CARE

- In cases with low C3 or C4 levels or low CH50, nonimmune complex causes of hypocomplementemia should be considered before making a definitive diagnosis of immune complex-mediated disease or genetic complement deficiencies.
- When using complement activity and complement factor levels to monitor disease activity in immune complex-mediated disorders, trends in test result values are more significant than single values. This is especially true in patients who are pregnant or who have concomitant inflammatory disorders, for whom a significant decrease in complement levels can signal increased disease activity, even if the complement levels are still within the normal range.

6 Immunoglobulins

ERRORS IN THE EVALUATION OF PROTEIN ELECTROPHORESIS

OVERVIEW

▶ Protein electrophoresis is a technique by which serum or urine proteins are separated by application of an electrical field to proteins loaded on a semi-solid matrix. The resolution varies by assay, but proteins typically resolve into five distinct regions, representing albumin and alpha-1, alpha-2, beta, and gamma globulins. The concentration of each band is determined by densitometry. Because the shapes and relative concentrations of each band differ in a variety of pathologic conditions, protein electrophoresis can be a useful adjunctive diagnostic test for many diseases. However, its primary purpose is the detection, measurement, and monitoring of monoclonal immunoglobulin generated by plasma cell neoplasms. Monoclonal immunoglobulins appear as a sharp spike, typically in the gamma regions on electrophoresis. This so-called "M spike" can be further analyzed by immunofixation electrophoresis, which defines the heavy and light chain constituents of this abnormal band so that they can be followed in subsequently collected specimens.

Case with Error

A 62-year-old man is diagnosed with plasma cell myeloma. Serum protein electrophoresis shows an M-spike composed of IgA lambda. He receives two cycles of standard chemotherapy, after which the response is assessed by repeat electrophoresis. When no M-spike is detected on this specimen, a complete response is declared and the patient receives an autologous stem cell transplant. However, he relapses with active disease just a few months after his transplant.

Explanation and Consequences

In this case, there was a failure to confirm a negative serum protein electrophoresis with immunofixation. Patients with minimal residual myeloma can have small M-spikes that are obscured by the normal serum protein bands. This is particularly problematic in patients with IgA myeloma. IgA species migrate at the upper end of the gamma region or in the beta region. A monoclonal IgA in the latter category can be easily obscured by the many normal proteins in the beta region.

If light chain immunofixation electrophoresis was performed in this case, a faint but distinct lambda band would have been detected in the beta region. Consequently, the patient would have been recategorized as having an incomplete response, and stem cell transplant would have been delayed in favor of further therapy. Instead, the patient was incorrectly classified and received a premature, and ultimately ineffective, transplant.

Case with Error

A 69-year-old woman presents with a history of fatigue and bone pain. Laboratory studies show elevated total protein with decreased albumin. Suspecting a plasma cell neoplasm, the physician orders serum protein electrophoresis. The blood is drawn into a serum separator tube, which is immediately centrifuged and sent to the laboratory. Electrophoresis reveals a spike at the border between the beta and gamma regions. To confirm the diagnosis, the patient receives a bone marrow biopsy. However, this shows no increase in plasma cells. Quantitative immunoglobulins are also normal.

Explanation and Consequences

In this case, the specimen for serum protein electrophoresis was improperly handled. Blood collected into serum separator tubes must be allowed to clot for at least 30 minutes after collection before centrifugation. Failure to do so will cause contamination of the serum with clotting proteins. In this case, the spike observed on protein electrophoresis was most likely fibrinogen from plasma that persisted in this poorly clotted specimen.

Besides fibrinogen, other protein bands can appear as prominent in certain clinical situations, mimicking an immunoglobulin M-spike. For example, in hemolytic anemia, there can be a prominent band that represents haptoglobin-hemoglobin complex. Similarly, C-reactive protein can be prominent in acute phase reactions, and transferrin can be increased in iron deficiency.

Misinterpretation of these prominent bands as M-spikes can be avoided in several ways. A positive protein electrophoresis should always be followed by immunofixation. Not only does this identify the monoclonal immunoglobulin species in positive cases, but it will be negative for the potentially confounding bands listed above. Immunofixation can also be performed for fibrinogen, allowing for its positive identification. Alternatively, the sample can be pretreated with thrombin, after which the fibrinogen band will disappear from electrophoresis. Finally, normal quantitative immunoglobulin levels, as were seen in this case, argue strongly against the presence of monoclonal immunoglobulin. Had these procedures been followed, the interfering fibrinogen would have been identified, preventing an invasive procedure for this patient.

Case with Error

A 56-year-old woman receives an autologous stem cell transplant for IgG-kappa plasma cell myeloma. Three months after transplant, serum protein electrophoresis is performed as surveillance for recurrent disease. Electrophoresis shows three distinct bands in the gamma region that are positive for kappa by immunofixation. Concerned for relapse, the hematologist performs a bone marrow biopsy that is negative for myeloma.

Explanation and Consequences

In this case, the kappa-positive bands in the gamma region were misinterpreted as a return of the patient's monoclonal IgG kappa. In fact, they represented oligoclonal bands. These are multiple distinct bands that often represent the emergence of an oligoclonal humoral immune response after transplantation. These multiple bands generally migrate differently than the patient's original M-spike, even if they are of the same light-chain species. However, it is possible by chance to see similarities in migration that can create confusion. In this case, misinterpretation of these oligoclonal bands as recurrence of the patient's previous M-spike led to an unnecessary bone marrow biopsy.

Case with Error

A 59-year-old man is found to have mild renal insufficiency on routine laboratory studies at his annual check-up. Serum protein electrophoresis is performed as part of the routine evaluation. No M-spike is observed, but densitometry shows a relative decrease in the gamma band. Six months later, the same patient presents with back pain. Radiologic studies show a compression fracture of a thoracic vertebra and multiple lytic bone lesions scattered throughout the axial skeleton. Bone marrow biopsy confirms a diagnosis of plasma cell myeloma. Urine studies show a significant quantity of Bence-Jones protein composed of kappa light chain.

Explanation and Consequences

In this case, a complete evaluation should have included both serum and urine protein electrophoresis. Approximately 20% of plasma cell myelomas produce only light chains with no heavy chain component. Because the light chains are rapidly filtered from the blood by the kidneys, they may not be detected on serum protein electrophoresis. However, a significant M-spike will be seen on urine protein electrophoresis.

In this case, an additional diagnostic clue for myeloma was a decrease in the gamma band. This indicates suppression of normal polyclonal immunoglobulin production that is typical of myeloma. Also, measurement of serum free light chains (see below) would have detected an abnormal ratio of free kappa to lambda light chains. Recognition of these signs and performance of urine protein electrophoresis would have led to earlier diagnosis and treatment of the patient's myeloma, likely preventing the morbidity that developed in the subsequent 6 months.

STANDARDS OF CARE

▨ Blood collected for serum analysis must be allowed to adequately clot prior to centrifugation and electrophoresis. Failure to do so may lead to contamination by plasma proteins, such as fibrinogen, that can confound interpretation of the serum protein electrophoresis.

- Immunofixation electrophoresis should be performed for any positive or suspicious band on electrophoresis to determine if the band represents immunoglobulin and to potentially characterize its identity for follow-up studies.
- Immunofixation, at least for light chains, should be performed on all follow-up studies to detect low levels of persistent monoclonal immunoglobulin.
- The presence of any abnormal bands should be carefully interpreted in the context of the patient history. A history of stem cell transplant, acute-phase reaction, hemolysis, or iron deficiency should be noted to aid in distinguishing bona fide M-spikes from oligoclonal bands and other confounding bands that can mimic M-spikes.
- In screening for myeloma, both serum and urine electrophoresis should be performed to aid in the detection of light chain-only myeloma.

RECOMMENDED READING

O'Connell TX, Horita TJ, Kasravi B. Understanding and interpreting serum protein electrophoresis. *Am Fam Physician.* 2005;71:105–112.

Vavricka SR, Burri E, Beglinger C, Degen L, Manz M. Serum protein electrophoresis: an underused but very useful test. *Digestion.* 2009;79:203–210.

Wahed A, Risin S. Issues with Immunology and Serology Testing. In: Dasgupta A, Sepulveda JL, eds. *Accurate Results in the Clinical Laboratory: A Guide to Error Detection and Correction.* Amsterdam, Netherlands: Elsevier; 2013:295–304.

ERRORS IN THE ANALYSIS OF FREE LIGHT CHAINS

OVERVIEW

> Despite equal stoichiometry of heavy and light chains in intact immunoglobulin, plasma cells produce more light chains than heavy chains. Consequently, free light chains circulate in the blood and are excreted into urine. Both kappa and lambda free light chains can be measured by nephelometry. Their absolute values and the ratio between kappa and lambda light chains can be used as surrogate markers for monoclonal immunoglobulin in the diagnosis and monitoring of plasma cell myeloma. However, because they are cleared by the kidney, caution must be exercised in the interpretation of these values in patients with renal insufficiency.

Case with Error

A 49-year-old man presents with renal insufficiency and proteinuria. As part of the evaluation to determine the cause of renal failure, serum protein electrophoresis and serum free light chains are ordered. The serum protein electrophoresis is abnormal with decreased albumin, but normal gamma globulin levels, and no apparent M-spike. However, the serum free light chains are increased, with an elevated ratio of kappa to lambda as follows:

	Result	Reference Range
Kappa free light chain	7.13 mg/dL	0.33–1.94 mg/dL
Lambda free light chain	2.61 mg/dL	0.57–2.63 mg/dL
Kappa:lambda ratio	2.7	0.26–1.65

Concerned that this may indicate a plasma cell disorder, the patient is referred to hematology for a bone marrow biopsy. However, the biopsy is negative for a clonal plasma cell population.

Explanation and Consequences

In this case, a kappa free light chain excess was interpreted as evidence of a monoclonal gammopathy. However, it is important to recognize that because serum free light chains are cleared by the kidney, they can be elevated in patients with renal insufficiency. In addition, there is a preference for retention of kappa light chains, such that the kappa:lambda light chain ratio is often elevated in renal disease. This can lead to misdiagnosis of monoclonal gammopathy.

The kappa light chain preference can lead to errors in the opposite direction as well. If a patient with monoclonal lambda light chain gammopathy has renal insufficiency, the preferential retention of kappa light chains can raise the kappa:lambda ratio into the normal range, masking the lambda light chain excess, and leading to a missed diagnosis.

In this case, the absence of an M-spike on protein electrophoresis was an important clue that the light chain ratio could be misleading. Of course, it could have been negative because the patient may have had light chain-only myeloma, but that would be detected by urine protein electrophoresis. Thus, it would have been better to order urine protein electrophoresis to confirm a monoclonal gammopathy before resorting to an invasive procedure like bone marrow biopsy.

STANDARDS OF CARE

- Serum free light chains must always be interpreted in the proper clinical context. In particular, elevated free light chains and high kappa:lambda ratios should be interpreted with caution in patients with renal insufficiency.
- Serum free light chains should not be evaluated independent of protein electrophoresis. While the light chain assays are a good screening tool, definitive diagnosis of monoclonal gammopathy requires the presence of an M-spike on serum and/or urine electrophoresis.

ERRORS IN THE ANALYSIS OF CRYOGLOBULINS

OVERVIEW

▶ Cryoglobulins are serum immunoglobulins that precipitate at temperatures lower than normal body temperature. They are classified as three different types. Type I cryoglobulins are single monoclonal immunoglobulins, often associated with B cell or plasma cell neoplasms. Type II cryoglobulins are mixtures of polyclonal and monoclonal immunoglobulins. Type III cryoglobulins are polyclonal IgM. Mixed cryoglobulins (types II and III) are often associated with chronic viral infections, typically hepatitis C. Precipitation of cryoglobulins in serum can activate complement, leading to an inflammatory vasculitis. Cryoglobulins are measured by allowing them to precipitate at 4°C, quantifying the volume of cryoglobulin (cryocrit) and analyzing the cryoglobulin content by protein electrophoresis.

Case with Error

A 45-year-old woman with a history of chronic hepatitis C infection and cirrhosis presents with frequent episodes of Raynaud's phenomenon. Concerned for cryoglobulinemia, her physician orders a cryocrit and cryoglobulin analysis. The specimen is drawn and transported to the laboratory at room temperature. No cryoglobulin is detected, and no treatment is initiated. Six months later, she presents to a different facility, now exhibiting fatigue, joint pain, and multiple purpuric skin lesions with ulceration on her lower limbs. A repeat analysis shows a positive cryocrit with type II cryoglobulins.

Explanation and Consequences

For the initial analysis in this case, the sample was handled incorrectly, causing a false–negative result. Because cryoglobulins precipitate at temperatures lower than 37°C, it is critical that the specimen be kept at 37°C from the time of collection, during transport and handling, and during centrifugation until the serum is separated and removed. In this case, the specimen was transported to the laboratory at room temperature, well below 37°C. This caused the cryoglobulins to precipitate prematurely, and they were subsequently centrifuged down with the red blood cells, removed from the serum, and lost prior to analysis. This preanalytical error caused a delay in definitive diagnosis and therapy.

Case with Error

A 69-year-old man with a long history of monoclonal gammopathy of undetermined significance (MGUS) presents to the emergency department with swelling of his left leg and is found to have a deep venous thrombosis. He is admitted to the hospital and started on intravenous heparin. During his initial evaluation, multiple small purpuric lesions were noted on both legs. Because of the history of monoclonal gammopathy, a consulting hematologist orders a cryocrit, which is positive.

Explanation and Consequences

The cryoglobulin analysis in this case was falsely positive due to the presence of heparin in the sample. Heparin creates complexes with serum proteins, particularly fibronectin, that precipitate in the cold. These precipitates will appear identical to cryoprecipitate on a cryocrit assay. This error could have been detected if the cryocrit assay had been followed by electrophoresis. This would have shown a single band that was negative by heavy and light chain immunofixation. This false-positive result could be significant if it prompted inappropriate treatment for cryoglobulinemia.

STANDARDS OF CARE

Samples drawn for cryoglobulin assays must be placed promptly in a 37°C water bath for transport, and then handled and centrifuged at 37°C within the laboratory. Samples should not be allowed to cool below 37°C until after centrifugation to prevent loss of precipitated cryoglobulins.

▨ Samples for cryoglobulin assays should not be drawn from a patient receiving intravenous heparin. Also, samples should be drawn from a peripheral vein, rather than from an intravenous line. If a sample must be drawn from an intravenous line, the first 10 mL of blood should be discarded prior to collection of the sample.

RECOMMENDED READING

Motyckova G, Murali M. Laboratory testing for cryoglobulins. *Am J Hematol.* 2011;86:500–502.

Shihabi ZK. Cryoglobulins: an important but neglected clinical test. *Ann Clin Lab Sci.* 2006;36:395–408.

Index